Diabetic Cookbook fo

100+ Simple & Healthy, Low-Sugar & Low-Carb Recipes for Type 2 Diabetes. 30-Day Diet Meal Plan for Time-Saving and Tasty Cooking

By GILLIAN RUELL

Table of contents

Contents

Introduction

In a world filled with conflicting information about health and nutrition, finding the right path to managing conditions like diabetes can feel like navigating a maze blindfolded. Having experienced the challenges and victories of living with diabetes myself, I understand the frustration and uncertainty that can come with this journey. But don't worry, dear reader, because this book holds the key to hope and clarity — a healthier and happier life.

For fifteen years, I have been on a quest to unlock the secrets of managing diabetes, not just for myself but for my loved ones as well. It all began with a diagnosis that rocked my world and forced me to confront the harsh reality of living with a chronic condition. But rather than fall to despair, I faced this challenge head-on, armed with a determination to take control of my health and well-being.

Through years of trial and error, I have honed my knowledge and expertise in diabetes management, drawing from scientific research and personal experience to develop effective strategies. I have walked the path you are embarking on now, and I am here to guide you every step of the way.

Through my experience, I have seen firsthand the transformative power of adopting a diabetes-friendly lifestyle, not just in my own life but in the lives of those I care about most. By helping my grandmothers and mother navigate the complexities of diabetes management, I have witnessed the vast benefits that small changes can reap from the wealth of knowledge and wisdom I have accumulated over the years, providing you with a focus on overall health and well-being.

Through this book, I aim to share practical tools and actionable strategies for managing diabetes and reclaiming health. From understanding the fundamentals of blood sugar management to mastering the art of meal planning, each chapter empowers you to make informed decisions about your health and well-being. Perhaps most importantly, this book is about more than managing diabetes—it's about transforming your life. By implementing the strategies outlined within these pages, you will improve your physical health and enhance your quality of life in ways you never thought possible. Imagine waking up each day feeling energized and empowered, knowing that you have the knowledge and tools to thrive despite the challenges that diabetes may present.

I invite you to join me on this journey of discovery, empowerment, and transformation. Together, we will navigate the complexities of diabetes management with courage, resilience, and unwavering determination. As we embark on this path together, remember you are not alone. I am here to support you every step of the way, offering guidance, encouragement, and expertise to help you through your journey to your health and wellness goals.

Now, without further ado, let us dive into the first chapter and begin our journey toward a healthier, happier future.

Understanding Types of Diabetes
What is Diabetes?

Diabetes occurs due to changes in the body's ability to process glucose, the primary energy source derived from carbohydrates in our diet. This alteration leads to a disturbance in the body's ability to regulate blood sugar levels (CDC, 2021). This imbalance arises due to inadequate insulin production or the body's inability to use insulin effectively.

In Type 1 Diabetes, the immune system, which is supposed to help fight germs, attacks and destroys cells of the pancreas cells that produce insulin. This means that individuals with type 1 diabetes rely on external insulin sources, usually through injections or insulin pumps, to keep their blood sugar regular. This type of diabetes is often seen in childhood or during adolescence. However, it is not restricted to any age.

Type 2 Diabetes occurs due to insulin resistance and inadequate insulin secretion. In this type, the body refuses to respond to insulin or doesn't produce enough to meet its needs. Type 2 diabetes is usually linked to lifestyle factors such as obesity, physical inactivity, and poor dietary habits. While it often develops in adulthood, its prevalence among children and adolescents is increasing, primarily due to rising rates of obesity.

Two others of diabetes that are not as common as the two above include gestational diabetes and prediabetes.

Gestational diabetes occurs during pregnancy when blood sugar levels rise higher than usual. It usually resolves after giving birth but can increase the risk of type 2 diabetes later in life.

Prediabetes, on the other hand, is a condition where blood sugar levels are higher than usual but not high enough to be classified as type 2 diabetes. It's a warning sign that someone is at risk of developing diabetes if they don't make lifestyle changes.

During the day, both gestational diabetes and prediabetes increase the likelihood of developing type 2 diabetes.

We will further discuss type 1 and type 2 diabetes below.

Both types of diabetes pose significant health risks if left unmanaged. Complications can include cardiovascular disease, kidney dysfunction, nerve damage, and vision impairment. Hence, it's paramount for individuals with diabetes to adopt comprehensive management strategies encompassing medication, dietary adjustments, regular physical activity, and vigilant monitoring of blood sugar levels.

Types of Diabetes

Diabetes manifests in different forms, each with its unique characteristics and management approaches. Let's explore the primary types.

Type 1 Diabetes:

Type 1 diabetes is like having a bodyguard who mistakenly attacks the good guys. In this case, the body's immune system, which is supposed to protect us from harmful invaders like bacteria and viruses, gets confused and starts attacking the pancreas. The pancreas is like a factory that produces insulin. This hormone transports sugar in the blood into our cells to give us energy. When the pancreas is under attack, it can't make enough insulin, and sugar piles up in the blood.

Management of Type 1 Diabetes involves a few key steps:

1. Insulin Injections or Pump: Since the body can't make adequate insulin, people with type 1 diabetes need insulin from outside sources. This can be done through injections using a needle and syringe or with an insulin pump like a tiny computerized device continuously delivering insulin throughout the day.

2. Monitoring Blood Sugar Levels: It is essential to monitor your blood sugar levels to manage type 1 diabetes effectively. This is usually done by pricking a finger to get a drop of blood and then using a glucose meter to measure the sugar level. It's like checking a car's fuel gauge to ensure enough gas for the journey.

3. Balancing Food and Insulin: Matching the right amount of food with the right amount of insulin is essential. Eating foods with carbohydrates, like bread and pasta, can cause a rapid rise in the amount of sugar in the blood. This makes it extremely important to adjust insulin doses accordingly. It's like a balancing act to keep blood sugar levels in check.

4. Regular Exercise: Staying active is beneficial for managing blood sugar levels in type 1 diabetes. Exercise can help increase insulin's effectiveness and lower blood sugar levels. It's like giving the body a boost to help it work better.

Type 2 Diabetes:

Type 2 diabetes is like having too many cars on the road and not enough traffic controllers. In this case, the body's traffic controllers, which are supposed to help sugar move from the blood into the cells, aren't working correctly. This can happen because the body becomes resistant to insulin or the pancreas can't make enough insulin to keep up with the demand.

Management of Type 2 Diabetes involves a few key steps:

Healthy Eating: This is another lifestyle modification essential for managing type 2 diabetes. This means choosing foods low in sugar and carbs, like fruits, vegetables, whole grains, and lean proteins. It's like giving the body the right fuel to keep it running smoothly.

Regular Exercise: Being active helps you maintain lower blood sugar levels and make your body more sensitive to insulin. You can keep it simple: playing basketball with friends, riding a bike, or walking. It's like giving the body a workout to keep it strong and healthy.

Medication: Sometimes, lifestyle changes alone aren't enough to manage type 2 diabetes. In these cases, doctors may prescribe medication to help lower blood sugar levels. These medications work in different ways, such as allowing the body to make more insulin or making the cells more sensitive to insulin. It's like adding extra help to get the job done.

Monitor Your Blood Sugar: One of the most important things to do almost daily is to check your blood sugar levels. A glucose meter can be used to do this regularly. It's like watching the road to ensure everything runs smoothly.

Symptoms of Diabetes

Diabetes can sometimes sneak up on us without showing any obvious signs. But there are some clues our bodies might give us to let us know that something's not quite right. Here are some common symptoms of diabetes:

Thirsty All the Time: Have you noticed that you're constantly thirsty, no matter how much water you drink? This could be a sign that your body is attempting to remove the excess sugar by making you pee more, which makes you thirsty.

Going to the Bathroom a Lot: If you need to pee more often than usual, especially at night, it might be a sign of diabetes. This happens because your body is trying to remove the excess glucose or sugar in your blood through your urine.

Feeling Tired: Do you always feel tired, even when you get enough sleep? Diabetes can make you feel exhausted because your body's cells aren't getting the energy they need from sugar.

Blurry vision is one of the many signs of diabetes. Excess blood sugar can cause the eye's lens to swell, reducing vision.

Slow Healing Wounds: Do cuts and bruises take longer than usual to heal? This could be a sign that your blood sugar levels are too high, which can slow down the body's ability to heal itself.

Unexplained Weight Loss: Losing weight without trying might sound like a dream, but it can be a sign of diabetes. When your body can't use sugar for energy, it starts burning fat and muscle, leading to weight loss.

The Role of Diet in Managing Diabetes

Diet plays a highly crucial role in managing diabetes. Think of your body as a car and food as its fuel. When you have diabetes, you need to be extra careful about the type and amount of fuel you put into your body to keep it running smoothly.

Here's how you can manage your diabetes through diet:

Choose Healthy Foods: Just like you want to put good-quality fuel into your car, you want to eat foods that are good for your body. This means choosing foods with low fat, sugar, and salt content but rich in nutrients like vitamins, minerals, and fiber. Good options include fruits, vegetables, whole grains, lean proteins (like chicken, fish, and beans), and healthy fats contained in avocados, seeds, nuts, and several other foods, which we will discuss in this book.

Watch Your Portions: It's not just about what you eat but how much you eat. Paying attention to portion sizes can go a long way to prevent overeating, which can cause spikes in blood sugar levels. Using smaller plates, measuring your food, and tracking serving sizes on food packages can help you control portions.

Cut Out Sugary Foods and Drinks: It is no surprise that these foods can spike sugar levels, so limiting them in your diet is essential. This includes candy, soda, fruit juice, and sweets. Instead, choose naturally sweet foods like fruits and limit sugary treats to occasional indulgences.

Eat and Snack at Regular Intervals: Going without food for a long time or skipping meals can cause your blood sugar levels to drop to dangerous levels. Eating frequent (not too many) meals, snacks, and intervals throughout the day is much better. This will help you maintain a more stable blood sugar level.

Balance Carbohydrates: Carbohydrates (carbs) are an essential energy source, but they also have the downside of causing blood sugar levels to rise. To manage diabetes, balancing your carb intake with other nutrients like protein and healthy fats is crucial. Go for complex carbs. Some of the few in this book include whole grains, fruits, and vegetables. These complex carbs don't cause drastic changes to your blood sugar levels.

Be Mindful of Timing: Your blood sugar levels can also be affected when you eat. Aim to spread your carb intake evenly. In the twenty-four hours of the day, avoid large meals just before bedtime, which can cause blood sugar levels to spike overnight.

Stay Hydrated: Staying well hydrated is one of the best things you can do for yourself. Sufficient water consumption is vital for maintaining good health and can assist in managing diabetes. Water is crucial for eliminating surplus sugar from the bloodstream and maintaining proper hydration levels, which is essential for supporting the body's basic functions. Remember, managing diabetes through diet is not about following a strict set of rules or depriving yourself. It's more about making and living more healthily. By paying attention to what you eat, watching your portions, and staying mindful of your body's signals, you can effectively manage your diabetes and live a happy, healthy life.

Tips for Healthy Cooking and Eating

Cooking and eating healthy doesn't have to be complicated, especially when managing diabetes. Here are some simple tips to help you make delicious and nutritious meals:

Fill Your Plate with Color: Consuming various colorful fruits and vegetables makes your diet visually appealing and offers a plethora of vitamins, minerals, and antioxidants that are beneficial to your health.

Go For Lean Proteins: Protein is the primary food class that helps build and repair body tissues. Lean protein sources such as chicken, turkey, fish, tofu, beans, and lentils are better for you. These protein sources contain less saturated fat and can give you a feeling of fullness and satisfaction.

Cook with Healthy Fats: Not all fats are bad for you. Healthy fats in nuts, avocados, seeds, and olive oil benefit heart health and help keep you full. Use these fats in moderation when cooking and preparing meals.

Limit Added Sugars: Added sugars can sneak into many processed foods and beverages, contributing to spikes in blood sugar levels. Limit your sugary foods and drinks intake and opt for naturally sweet options like fruits.

Monitor Your Portions: Portion control is essential for managing diabetes and maintaining a healthy weight. Use smaller plates and bowls, measure serving sizes, and be mindful of portions when eating out.

Cook at Home: Cooking at home gives you more control over your ingredients and cooking methods. Try to prepare meals at home as much as possible, using fresh, whole ingredients.

Plan Ahead: Planning your meals and snacks can prevent you from breaking your diet and ensure you eat appropriately. Take weekly time to plan your meals, make a grocery list, and prep ingredients.

Stay Hydrated: Although this has been covered before, it is something that you should always remember. Your daily aim should be to drink at least eight glasses of water and more if you're active or live in a hot climate.

Chapter 1

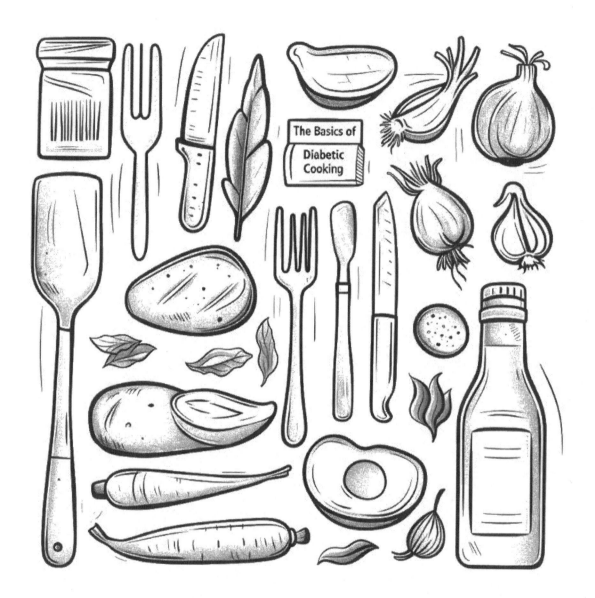

The Basics of Diabetic Cooking

Understanding Carbohydrates: The Good and The Bad

Carbohydrates, or "carbs" for short, are like the fuel that powers our bodies. They provide us the energy to do everything we love, like playing sports, studying, and hanging out with friends (Harvard Health Publishing, 2021). But not all carbs are created equal. Some are good for us, while others can cause problems, especially if you have diabetes.

Let's break it down:

The Good Carbs:

Good carbs are like slow-burning fuel that keeps us going throughout the day without causing big spikes in blood sugar. These are often found in foods high in fiber, like fruits, vegetables, whole grains, and legumes (like beans and lentils). Good carbs take longer for our bodies to break down, providing a steady energy source and helping us feel full and satisfied.

Examples of good carbs include

Fruits: Apples, oranges, berries, bananas

Vegetables: Spinach, broccoli, carrots, bell peppers

Whole Grains: Brown rice, quinoa, oats, whole wheat bread

Legumes: Chickpeas, black beans, lentils

The Bad Carbs:

Bad carbs are like quick-burning fuel that gives us energy but leaves us tired and hungry soon after. They are often found in processed foods, including white rice, white bread, sugary snacks, and sweetened beverages. Bad carbs cause our blood sugar levels to spike quickly, which can be dangerous, especially for people with diabetes.

Examples of bad carbs include:

Sugary Snacks: Candy, cookies, cake, pastries

Sugary Beverages: Soda, fruit juice, energy drinks

Refined Grains: Pasta, white rice, and white bread are made from white flour

Processed Foods: Chips, crackers, and packaged snacks

So, how can we make sure we're eating more of the good carbs and less of the bad ones?

Tips for Choosing Good Carbs:

Go for Whole Foods: Whenever possible, choose whole, unprocessed foods. These foods are often higher in fiber and nutrients and lower in added sugars and refined grains.

Read Labels: Check the nutrition labels on packaged foods to see how much fiber and sugar they contain. Aim for foods with higher fiber content and lower sugar content.

Swap Out Bad Carbs for Good Ones: Instead of white bread, try whole wheat bread. Instead of white rice, try brown rice or quinoa.

Watch Your Portions: Even good carbs can lead to spikes in blood sugar levels if you overeat. Watch your portion sizes and ensure your meals balance carbs, protein, and healthy fats.

By understanding the difference between good and bad carbs, you can make smarter choices about what you eat and better manage your diabetes.

The Importance of Low-Sugar and Low-Carb Eating

When it comes to managing diabetes, what you eat matters a lot. That's where low-sugar and low-carb eating comes into play. Let's break it down in simple terms:

What are Sugars and Carbs?

As I said, sugars and carbohydrates are sweet and starchy parts of food that give us energy. Sugars are found in candy, soda, and desserts, while carbs are in bread, pasta, and rice. When we eat these foods, they turn into sugar in our bodies, which can cause our blood sugar levels to rise.

The Problem with Too Much Sugar and Carbs:

Having too much sugar and carbs in our diet can be a problem, especially if you have diabetes. When our blood sugar levels get too high, it can cause many health issues, like feeling tired, thirsty, and needing to pee a lot. Over time, constantly elevated high blood sugar can lead to severe conditions like heart disease, kidney problems, and eye damage.

The Benefits of Low-Sugar and Low-Carb Eating:

Eating foods low in sugar and carbs can help stabilize your blood sugar levels and reduce the risk of these complications. Here's why it's important:

Stable Blood Sugar Levels: Foods that are low in sugar and carbs cause smaller spikes in blood sugar levels, which means our bodies can handle them better. This helps keep our energy levels steady throughout the day and prevents those highs and lows that can make us feel yucky.

Better Weight Management: Foods that are low in sugar and carbs are often lower in calories, which keeps us from being overweight. You may ask why this is important. The reason is simply that it is more difficult to manage diabetes when one is overweight. It also increases the likelihood of complications like the ones mentioned above happening.

Improved Insulin Sensitivity: Eating fewer carbs can increase the sensitivity of our body cells to insulin. This means our bodies can use insulin more effectively, which helps our body regulate blood sugar more effectively and those who may have insulin resistance.

Tips for Low-Sugar and Low-Carb Eating:

- Choose whole, unprocessed foods like fruits, vegetables, lean proteins, and whole grains.
- Limit sugary snacks and drinks like candy, soda, and fruit juice.
- Opt for high-fiber carbs like brown rice, quinoa, and whole wheat bread.
- Pay attention to portion sizes and aim for balance in your meals.
- Reading food labels can help you detect the added sugars and hidden carbs it contains.

Sugar Substitutes: Sweetening the Healthy Way

Sugar substitutes are magic ingredients that make our food taste sweet without adding extra sugar. They can be better alternatives for people with diabetes or those who want to watch their sugar consumption. Let's learn more about them:

What are Sugar Substitutes?

Sugar substitutes are ingredients that sweeten foods and drinks without adding regular sugar. They come in many different forms, including:

Artificial Sweeteners: These are made in a lab and are much sweeter than sugar, so you only need a bit to sweeten your food or drink. Examples include aspartame (found in diet soda), sucralose (found in Splenda), and saccharin (found in Sweet'N Low).

Natural Sweeteners: These are made from plants and are often less processed than artificial sweeteners. Examples include stevia (made from the leaves of the stevia plant), monk fruit extract (made from the fruit of the monk fruit plant), and erythritol (a sugar alcohol found in fruits and vegetables).

Why Use Sugar Substitutes?

There are a few reasons why someone might choose to use sugar substitutes:

Lower in Calories: Sugar substitutes are often lower in calories than regular sugar, which can help people trying to watch their weight.

Doesn't Raise Blood Sugar Levels: Many sugar substitutes don't raise blood sugar levels the way that regular sugar does, making them a good option for people with diabetes.

Helps Reduce Sugar Intake: Using sugar substitutes can help reduce our overall sugar intake, which is essential for our health.

Tips for Using Sugar Substitutes:

Start Small: Some sugar substitutes are much sweeter than sugar, so you only need a bit to sweeten your food or drink. Start with a small amount and add more if needed.
Experiment: There are many different types of sugar substitutes, so feel free to experiment and find the ones you like best.

Read Labels: Some products labeled "sugar-free" may still contain sugar substitutes, so reading the ingredients list is essential to know what you're getting.

Be Mindful of Side Effects: Certain sugar substitutes may cause digestive issues or other side effects, so it's essential to pay attention to how your body reacts.

Sugar Substitutes in Action:
- Add a packet of stevia to your morning coffee instead of sugar.
- Use monk fruit extract to sweeten your oatmeal or yogurt.
- Bake with erythritol instead of regular sugar in your favorite recipes.
- Using sugar substitutes instead of regular sugar allows you to enjoy sweet treats while keeping your blood sugar levels in check.

Portion Control: How Much to Eat
Portion control is like ensuring you don't eat too much or too little. It's about finding the right balance to enjoy your food while caring for your body. Here's why it's important and some tips to help you do it:

Why is Portion Control Important?
Eating the right amount of food is essential for many reasons:

Helps Manage Weight: Overeating can lead to weight gain while eating too little can lead to weight loss. Finding the correct portion sizes can help you maintain a healthy weight.

Controls Blood Sugar Levels: Overindulging in carbs or sugary treats can cause a quick surge in blood sugar levels, potentially endangering individuals, especially those with diabetes. Portion control can help keep your blood sugar levels stable.

Prevents Overeating: Eating more than we can makes us feel uncomfortable and sluggish. Portion control helps avoid overeating and keeps us feeling good after meals.

Tips for Portion Control:

Use Visual Cues: Use your hand or everyday objects to estimate portion sizes. For example, a serving of meat should be about the size of your palm, a serving of carbs (like rice or pasta) should be the size of your fist, and a serving of fats (like butter or oil) should be the size of your thumb.

Read Labels: Pay attention to serving sizes on food labels to ensure you eat only what you need. Estimating how much we eat is easy, so reading labels can help us stay on track.

Use Smaller Plates: Smaller plates and bowls can deceive your mind into believing you've consumed more food than you have, resulting in satisfaction with smaller serving sizes.

Listen to Your Body: Be mindful of your body's signals of hunger and fullness. Consume food when you feel hungry and cease eating when you're satisfied, regardless of whether food remains on your plate.

Slow Down: Taking time to eat allows your body to recognize satiety cues, reducing the likelihood of overeating. Pause between bites, chew your food thoughtfully and enjoy the flavors with each mouthful.

By practicing portion control, you can enjoy your favorite foods while caring for your health. It's all about finding the right balance for you and your body.

Reading Food Labels: What to Look For?

Reading food labels is like decoding a secret message that tells you what's really in your food. It's an essential skill for making healthy choices and managing your diabetes. Here's what to look for when reading food labels:

1. Serving Size:

The serving size provides all you need to know about nutrition in a food. Pay attention to this because the rest of the information on the label is for one serving. You must adjust the numbers if you eat more or less than the serving size.

2. Total Carbohydrates:

This tells you how many carbs are in one serving of the food. Carbs include sugars, fiber, and starches. For people with diabetes, keeping track of the total carbs to help manage blood sugar levels is essential.

3. Added Sugars:

Added sugars are extra sweeteners added to food products during manufacturing or cooking. They can hide in foods you wouldn't expect, like sauces, dressings, and snacks. Monitoring added sugars can help you make healthier choices and avoid unnecessary sugar intake.

4. Fiber:

Fibre is a type of carbohydrate that's good for you. It helps keep you full, aids digestion, and controls blood sugar levels. Look for fiber-rich foods to support your overall health and diabetes management.

5. Sodium:

Sodium is another name for salt, and it's found in many processed and packaged foods. Excessive sodium intake can elevate the likelihood of developing high blood pressure and various other health complications. Try to choose lower-sodium foods to keep your heart healthy.

6. Ingredients List:

The ingredients list tells you what's in the food, starting with the most abundant ingredient and ending with the least. This list is essential to avoid specific ingredients such as added sugars or unhealthy fats.

By learning how to read food labels and understanding what to look for, you can make informed choices about your foods and better manage your diabetes.

Dedicate some time to thoroughly review labels and opt for foods that promote your health and overall well-being.

Chapter 2

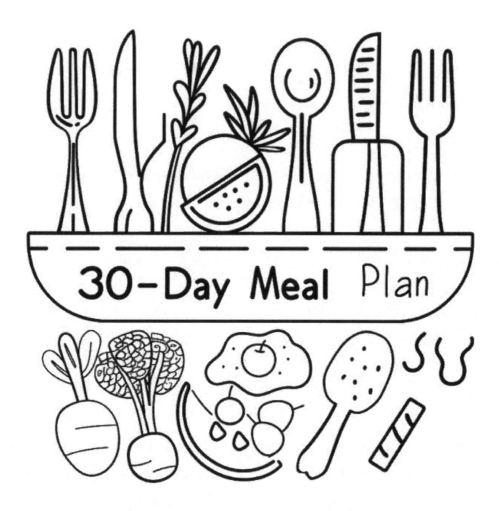

30-Day Meal Plan

Introducing the "30-Day Meal Plan" chapter, your roadmap to delicious and nutritious meals designed specifically for managing diabetes. Learn how to plan your meals effectively, follow a comprehensive 30-day calendar with daily meal plans, streamline your grocery shopping with weekly lists, and master meal-prepping for time-saving success.

How to Plan Your Meals

Planning your meals is like drawing up a map for your food journey. It helps you eat the right things at the correct times to keep your body happy and healthy. Here's how to do it:

1. Set Your Goals: Think about what you want to achieve with your meals. Do you want to manage your blood sugar levels better? Lose weight? Feel more energized? Your goals will guide your meal-planning decisions.

2. Know Your Portions: Understanding portion sizes is vital to balanced eating. Use tools like measuring cups, spoons, and your hand to gauge appropriate serving sizes for different foods.

3. Choose Balanced Meals: Aim to include a mix of carbohydrates, protein, and healthy fats in each meal. Carbs provide energy, protein helps build and repair muscles, and fats keep you feeling full and satisfied.

4. Plan Ahead: Take some time each week to plan your meals for the upcoming days. Look at your calendar for your events or commitments and plan meals accordingly. This can prevent unnecessary last-minute stress and unhealthy food choices.

5. Get Creative: Feel free to try new foods and recipes. Experiment with different ingredients, flavors, and cooking methods to keep your meals exciting and enjoyable.

6. Consider Convenience: When planning meals, consider your schedule and lifestyle. Choose quick and easy recipes to prepare on busy days and save more elaborate meals when you have more time.

7. Use Resources:

Use cookbooks, online recipes, and meal-planning apps to generate meal ideas and recipes. Many resources are available to inspire and support you on your meal-planning journey. Meal planning doesn't have to be complicated—take it one meal at a time and do what works best for you.

30-Day Calendar with Daily Meal Plan

Below is a simple 30-day meal plan to guide your eating habits. Each day includes breakfast, lunch, dinner, and snacks, designed to provide balanced nutrition while managing diabetes. Feel free to adjust portion sizes and substitute ingredients depending on what you want.

The table below is an example of a 30-day calendar daily meal plan you can follow. You can also make adjustments or create a new one following the same template.

Day	Breakfast	Lunch	Dinner	Snacks
1	Oatmeal with fruit	Turkey Sandwich	Grilled chicken	Apple slices with nut butter
2	Greek yogurt with honey	Quinoa salad	Salmon with roasted vegetables	Carrot sticks with hummus
3	Scrambled eggs with spinach	Chicken stir-fry	Lentil soup	Mixed nuts
4	Whole grain toast with avocado	Tuna salad	Beef stir-fry	Cottage cheese with berries
5	Smoothie with banana and spinach	Veggie wrap	Baked fish with quinoa	Yogurt with granola
6	Pancakes with berries	Grilled cheese	Turkey chili	Celery sticks with peanut butter
7	Breakfast burrito	Chicken Caesar salad	Veggie lasagna	Cheese and whole grain crackers
8	Overnight oats	Veggie wrap	Stir-fried tofu	Sliced cucumber with tzatziki
9	Fruit salad	Lentil soup	Baked Chicken	Rice cakes with almond butter
10	Whole grain cereal with milk	Quinoa salad	Beef tacos	Trail mix
11	Egg muffins	Turkey Sandwich	Grilled salmon	Apple slices with cheese

Day	Breakfast	Lunch	Dinner	Snacks
12	Smoothie bowl with granola	Chicken Caesar salad	Veggie stir-fry	Yogurt with mixed berries
13	Breakfast smoothie	Quinoa bowl	Turkey meatballs	Carrot sticks with hummus
14	Avocado toast	Lentil soup	Baked fish	Greek yogurt with honey
15	Scrambled eggs with veggies	Veggie wrap	Beef stir-fry	Mixed nuts
16	Whole grain waffles	Greek salad	Chicken curry	Cottage cheese with fruit
17	Yogurt parfait	Turkey chili	Veggie lasagna	Cheese and crackers
18	Banana pancakes	Chicken stir-fry	Baked tofu	Celery sticks with peanut butter
19	Breakfast burrito	Quinoa salad	Grilled chicken	Rice cakes with almond butter
20	Oatmeal with nuts and berries	Tuna salad	Beef tacos	Trail mix
21	Smoothie with spinach and banana	Chicken Caesar salad	Veggie stir-fry	Apple slices with cheese
22	Greek yogurt with granola	Lentil soup	Baked salmon	Yogurt with mixed berries
23	Whole grain toast with avocado	Veggie wrap	Turkey meatballs	Carrot sticks with hummus
24	Fruit salad	Chicken Caesar salad	Beef stir-fry	Cottage cheese with fruit

Day	Breakfast	Lunch	Dinner	Snacks
25	Scrambled eggs with spinach	Quinoa bowl	Veggie lasagna	Mixed nuts
26	Smoothie bowl with granola	Lentil soup	Chicken curry	Cheese and crackers
27	Breakfast smoothie	Greek salad	Baked tofu	Celery sticks with peanut butter
28	Avocado toast	Turkey chili	Veggie stir-fry	Rice cakes with almond butter
29	Egg muffins	Chicken stir-fry	Grilled salmon	Trail mix
30	Whole grain waffles	Quinoa salad	Baked Chicken	Apple slices with nut butter

Weekly Shopping Lists

Weekly shopping lists are like your grocery game plan—they help you get everything you need for your meals without forgetting anything. Here's how to make and use them:

1. Make a Plan:

Before you head to the store, review your meal plan for the week. Note all the ingredients needed for each meal, including main ingredients, spices, and pantry staples.

2. Check Your Pantry:

Take a quick inventory of what you already have in your pantry, fridge, and freezer. This will help you avoid duplicates and ensure you only buy what you need.

3. Organize Your List:

Group your shopping list by categories: produce, dairy, proteins, and pantry items. This will make it easier to navigate the store and ensure you get everything.

4. Stick to Your Budget:

Decide how much you want to spend on groceries for the week, and stick to it. When you plan your meals ahead of time, you avoid buying impulsively and stay within your budget.

5. Be Flexible:

While having a plan is good, it's also important to be flexible. If you can't find a particular ingredient or it's too expensive, look for alternatives or adjust your meal plan accordingly.

Sample Shopping List:

Produce:

- Spinach
- Broccoli
- Carrots
- Bell peppers
- Apples
- Bananas
- Oranges
- Tomatoes
- Avocado

Dairy:

- Greek yoghurt
- Eggs
- Milk
- Cheese

Proteins:

- Chicken breasts
- Salmon fillets
- Lean ground turkey
- Tofu
- Beans (canned or dried)

Grains:

- Whole grain bread
- Brown rice
- Quinoa
- Whole wheat pasta

Pantry Staples:

- Olive oil
- Balsamic vinegar
- Spices (salt, pepper, garlic powder, onion powder, paprika)
- Canned tomatoes
- Chicken broth
- Oats
- Nuts and seeds
- Whole grain cereal

Snacks:

- Mixed nuts
- Hummus
- Whole grain crackers
- Rice cakes
- Trail mix
- Nut butter

Beverages:

- Water
- Herbal tea
- Coffee
- Unsweetened almond milk

Frozen Foods:

- Frozen berries
- Frozen vegetables
- Frozen shrimp

<u>Remember</u> to check your list before heading to the store and mark off items as you go. This will help you stay organized and ensure you remember everything. With a well-planned shopping list, you'll be ready to tackle your weekly grocery shopping easily.

Tips for Meal-Prepping and Time-Saving

Meal-prepping and time-saving tips are like magic tricks that help you spend less time in the kitchen and more time enjoying your meals. Here are some easy tips to get you started:

1. Plan Ahead:

Take some time at the beginning of the week to plan your meals and snacks. This will ensure that everything is orderly and avoid last-minute stress when it comes time to cook.

2. Cook in Batches:

Cooking in batches means making larger quantities of food at once and storing leftovers for later. This saves time because you only have to cook once but can enjoy multiple meals.

3. Use Your Freezer:

Your freezer is your best friend, especially when it comes to meal-prepping. Freeze leftovers, soups, stews, and casseroles in individual portions for quick and easy weekly meals.

4. Prep Ingredients in Advance:

To streamline your cooking process, chop vegetables, marinate meats, and prepare grains in advance. Prepped ingredients make it easier to throw together a meal quickly.

5. Invest in Time-Saving Tools:

Tools like a slow cooker, Instant Pot, or air fryer can help you cook meals faster with minimal effort. They're great for busy days when you only have a little time to spend in the kitchen.

6. Keep it Simple:

It is always better to cook simple recipes with fewer ingredients and shorter cooking times. You don't need fancy or complicated meals to eat well — sometimes, the simplest dishes are the most delicious.

7. Double Up on Recipes:

When you find a recipe you love, double or triple it and freeze the extra portions for later, this way, you'll always have a quick and easy meal.

8. Set Aside Time for Meal Prep:

Schedule dedicated time each week for meal prep. This could be on a Sunday afternoon or whatever day works best for you. Treat it like an appointment and prioritize it in your schedule.

9. Get the Whole Family Involved:

Meal-prepping can be a fun family activity! Get everyone involved in chopping vegetables, assembling meals, and packing lunches. It's a great way to spend quality time together and teach kids valuable cooking skills.

10. Don't Forget About Convenience Foods:

There's no shame in using convenience foods from time to time. Pre-packaged salads, pre-cooked grains, and rotisserie chicken can be lifesavers on busy days when you need a quick and easy meal option.

Adding these meal-prepping and time-saving tips to your routine will reduce your stress about what to eat and allow you to enjoy delicious and nutritious meals with your loved ones more.

Chapter 3

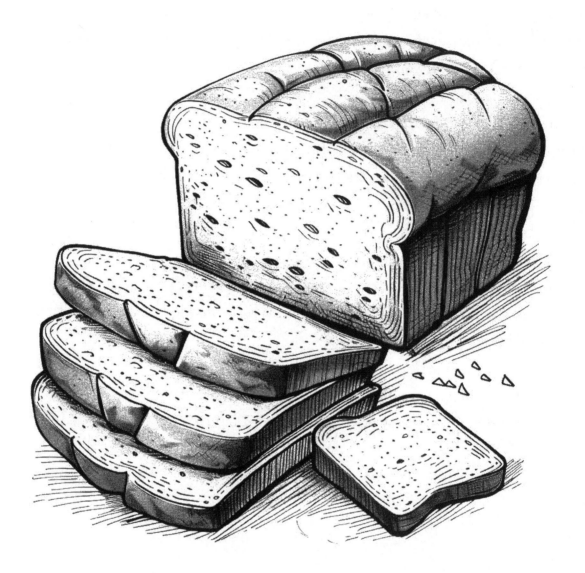

Low-carb bread recipes

These mouthwatering low-carb bread recipes will keep your blood sugar up long. Whether you're craving a hearty sandwich, a savory snack, or a tasty side dish, these recipes have covered you. These simple ingredients and easy-to-follow steps will help you make delicious homemade bread to manage your carb intake without sacrificing flavor. Say goodbye to store-bought bread and hello to wholesome, homemade goodness.

Simple Almond Flour Bread

 12 SLICES | PREP TIME: 10 MIN | COOK TIME: 40-45 MIN

INGREDIENTS

- 2 cups almond flour
- 4 large eggs
- 1/4 cup melted butter
- 1 teaspoon baking powder
- 1/2 teaspoon salt

NUTRITIONS

Calories Per Serving: 150 calories

Protein: 6 grams per slice.

Fat: 14 grams per slice.

Carbohydrates: 3 grams per slice.

DIRECTIONS

1. Preheat your oven to 350°F (175°C) or its equivalent. Grease or line a loaf pan with butter or parchment paper.
2. Blend the almond flour, baking powder, and salt in a large mixing bowl until thoroughly combined.
3. Whisk together the eggs and melted butter in a separate bowl until they form a smooth mixture.
4. Mix the wet and dry ingredients, stirring until a smooth batter forms.
5. Evenly transfer the batter into the prepared loaf pan.
6. Bake for 40-45 minutes until the bread is golden brown and a toothpick inserted into the center comes clean.
7. Allow the bread to cool in the pan for 10 minutes, then transfer it to a wire rack to completely cool. Once cooled, slice and serve.

Savory Zucchini Bread

 12 SLICES | PREP TIME: 15 MIN | COOK TIME: 50-55 MIN

INGREDIENTS

- 2 cups grated zucchini
- 2 cups almond flour
- 4 large eggs
- 1/4 cup olive oil
- 1 teaspoon baking powder
- 1/2 teaspoon garlic powder
- 1/2 teaspoon dried basil
- Salt and pepper to taste

NUTRITIONS

Calories Per Serving: 130 calories

Protein: 5 grams per slice.

Fat: 11 grams per slice.

Carbohydrates: 4 grams per slice.

DIRECTIONS

1. Preheat your oven to 350°F (175°C). Prepare a loaf pan by greasing it with butter or lining it with parchment paper.
2. Combine the grated zucchini, almond flour, baking powder, garlic powder, dried basil, salt, and pepper in a large mixing bowl.
3. Whisk together the eggs and olive oil in another bowl until well combined.
4. Pour the egg mixture into the dry ingredients and stir until fully incorporated.
5. Spread the batter evenly into the prepared loaf pan.
6. Bake for 50-55 minutes until the bread is firm to the touch and a toothpick inserted into the center comes out clean.
7. Let the bread cool in the pan for 10 minutes, then transfer it to a wire rack to cool completely. Slice and serve.

Herbed Cheese and Seed Bread

 12 SLICES | PREP TIME: 20 MIN | COOK TIME: 55-60 MIN

INGREDIENTS

- 2 cups almond flour
- 1/4 cup grated Parmesan cheese
- 1/4 cup shredded mozzarella cheese
- 4 large eggs
- 1/4 cup melted butter
- 1 teaspoon baking powder
- 1 tablespoon mixed seeds (such as sesame seeds, poppy seeds, and sunflower seeds)

NUTRITIONS

Calories Per Serving: 150 calories

Protein: 6 grams per slice.

Fat: 14 grams per slice.

Carbohydrates: 3 grams per slice.

DIRECTIONS

1. Preheat your oven to 350°F (175°C). Prepare
2. a loaf pan by greasing it with butter or lining it with parchment paper.
3. Combine the almond flour, grated Parmesan cheese, shredded mozzarella cheese, baking powder, mixed seeds, dried Italian herbs, salt, and pepper in a large mixing bowl.
4. In another bowl, beat the eggs and melted butter until well combined.
5. Pour the egg mixture into the dry ingredients and stir until the batter is smooth.
6. Transfer the batter to the prepared loaf pan and spread it out evenly.
7. Bake for 55-60 minutes until the bread is golden brown and a toothpick inserted into the center comes clean.
8. Allow the bread to cool in the pan for 10 minutes before transferring it to a wire rack to cool completely. Slice and serve.

Chapter 4

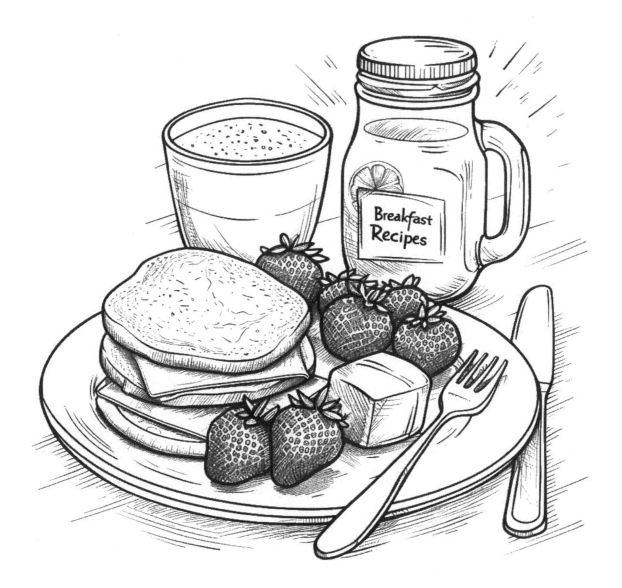

Breakfast Recipes

Welcome to the Breakfast Recipes chapter, where we'll explore various delicious and nutritious ways to start your day. Whether you prefer sweet or savory, quick and easy, or leisurely brunches, we've got you covered with recipes that are not only satisfying but also blood sugar-friendly. Say goodbye to boring breakfasts and hello to a morning routine that sets you up for success!

Overnight Oats

 1 SERVING | PREP TIME: 5 MIN | COOK TIME: OVERNIGHT

INGREDIENTS

- 1/2 cup old-fashioned oats
- 1/2 cup unsweetened almond milk
- 1/4 cup Greek yogurt
- 1 tablespoon chia seeds
- 1/2 teaspoon vanilla extract
- 1/2 cup mixed berries (such as strawberries, blueberries, and raspberries)
- 1 tablespoon chopped nuts (such as almonds or walnuts)
- 1 tablespoon honey or maple syrup (optional)
- 1 teaspoon dried Italian herbs (such as oregano, basil, and thyme)
- Salt and pepper to taste

NUTRITIONS
Calories Per Serving: 250 calories

Protein: 9 grams

Fat: 10 grams

Carbohydrates: 37

DIRECTIONS

1. In a container, combine oats, almond milk, Greek yogurt, chia seeds, and vanilla extract.
2. Stir well to combine all ingredients.
3. Add mixed berries and chopped nuts on top.
4. Drizzle honey or maple syrup on top if desired.
5. Cover and refrigerate overnight.
6. In the morning, stir the oats and enjoy cold or hot food in the microwave, if desired.

Spinach and Feta Breakfast Wrap

 1 WRAP

 PREP TIME: 5 MIN

 COOK TIME: 5 MIN

INGREDIENTS

- 1 whole grain tortilla
- 2 large eggs, scrambled
- 1/4 cup chopped spinach
- 2 tablespoons crumbled feta cheese
- Salt and pepper to taste

DIRECTIONS

1. Heat a non-stick skillet over medium heat and lightly coat it with cooking spray.
2. Warm the tortilla in the skillet for about 30 seconds on each side.
3. In a separate bowl, scramble the eggs and season with salt and pepper.
4. Cook chopped spinach in the skillet until wilted.
5. Pour the scrambled eggs over the spinach and cook until set.
6. Sprinkle crumbled feta cheese over the eggs and spinach.
7. Once the cheese has melted, transfer the mixture to the warmed tortilla.
8. Fold the sides of the tortilla over the filling to create a wrap.
9. Serve immediately

NUTRITIONS

Calories Per Serving: 300 calories

Protein: 20 grams

Fat: 13 grams

Carbohydrates: 23 gram

Peanut Butter Banana Smoothie

 1 SMOOTHIE | PREP TIME: 5 MIN | COOK TIME: 5 MIN

INGREDIENTS

- 1 ripe banana
- 1 tablespoon natural peanut butter
- 1/2 cup unsweetened almond milk
- 1/4 cup Greek yogurt
- 1 tablespoon honey (optional)
- Ice cubes

DIRECTIONS

1. Remove the banana peel and put the fruit in a blender.
2. Add peanut butter, almond milk, Greek yogurt, honey, and ice cubes to the blender.
3. Blend until smooth and creamy.
4. Pour into a glass and serve immediately.

NUTRITIONS

Calories Per Serving: 250 calories

Protein: 10 grams

Fat: 11 grams

Carbohydrates: 35 grams

Smoked Salmon and Cream Cheese Bagel

 1 BAGEL | PREP TIME: 5 MIN | COOK TIME: 5 MIN

INGREDIENTS

- 1 whole grain bagel, sliced and toasted
- 2 tablespoons low-fat cream cheese
- 2 ounces smoked salmon
- Thinly sliced red onion
- Capers

DIRECTIONS

1. Evenly spread cream cheese on both halves of the toasted bagel.
2. Place smoked salmon on one half of the bagel
3. Top the salmon with thinly sliced red onion and capers.
4. Cover with
5. the other half of the bagel to create a sandwich.
6. Serve immediately.

NUTRITIONS
Calories Per Serving: 300 calories

Protein: 17 grams

Fat: 9 grams

Carbohydrates: 33 grams

Veggie Omelette

 1 OMELETTE | PREP TIME: 5 MIN | COOK TIME: 5 MIN

INGREDIENTS

- 2 large eggs
- 1/4 cup chopped bell peppers
- 1/4 cup chopped onions
- 1/4 cup chopped spinach
- 1 tablespoon olive oil
- Salt and pepper to taste

NUTRITIONS

Calories Per Serving: 200 calories

Protein: 14 grams

Fat: 13 grams

Carbohydrates: 5 grams

DIRECTIONS

1. Beat the eggs in a bowl until thoroughly mixed—season with salt and pepper.
2. Heat olive oil in a non-stick skillet over medium heat.
3. Sauté chopped vegetables in the skillet until tender.
4. Pour the beaten eggs over the cooked vegetables.
5. Cook for 2-3 minutes until the edges start to set. Use a spatula to gently lift the edges and allow the uncooked eggs to flow underneath.
6. Once the eggs are set, fold the omelet in half and cook for another 1-2 minutes until fully cooked.
7. Slide the omelet onto a plate and serve hot.

Greek Yogurt Parfait

 1 PARFAIT | PREP TIME: 5 MIN | COOK TIME: 5 MIN

INGREDIENTS

- 1/2 cup plain Greek yogurt
- 1/4 cup mixed berries (such as strawberries, blueberries, and raspberries)
- 1 tablespoon chopped nuts (such as almonds or walnuts)
- 1 tablespoon honey (optional)

DIRECTIONS

1. Layer Greek yogurt, mixed berries, and chopped nuts in a glass or bowl.
2. Drizzle honey on top if desired.
3. Serve immediately and enjoy!

NUTRITIONS

Calories Per Serving: 150 calories

Protein: 10 grams

Fat: 5 grams

Carbohydrates: 10 grams

Avocado Toast

 1 TOAST | PREP TIME: 5 MIN | COOK TIME: 5 MIN

INGREDIENTS

- 1 slice whole grain bread, toasted
- 1/2 ripe avocado
- 1 teaspoon lemon juice
- Pinch of salt and pepper
- Optional toppings: sliced tomatoes, red pepper flakes, or a poached egg

DIRECTIONS

1. Mash the avocado with lemon juice, salt, and pepper in a bowl.
2. Spread the mashed avocado evenly on the toasted bread slice.
3. If desired, top with sliced tomatoes, red pepper flakes, or a poached egg.
4. Serve immediately.

NUTRITIONS

Calories Per Serving:

200 calories

Protein: 3 grams.

Fat: 15 grams.

Carbohydrates: 24 grams

Vegetable Breakfast Hash

 2 SERVINGS | PREP TIME: 10 MIN | COOK TIME: 15 MIN

INGREDIENTS

- 1 tablespoon olive oil
- 1 small sweet potato, diced
- 1/2 cup diced bell peppers
- 1/4 cup diced onions
- 1/4 cup diced zucchini
- 2 large eggs
- Salt and pepper to taste
- Optional toppings: salsa, avocado slices, chopped cilantro

DIRECTIONS

1. Pour olive oil into a skillet and heat it on medium heat
2. Cook diced sweet potato until slightly softened, about 5 minutes.
3. Add diced bell peppers, onions, and zucchini, and cook until the vegetables are soft, about 5-7 minutes.
4. Make two wells in the vegetable mixture and crack an egg into each.
5. Season eggs with salt and pepper.
6. Cover the skillet and leave to cook for about 5-7 minutes or until eggs are done to your liking, for a runny yolk.
7. Serve hot with optional toppings if desired.

NUTRITIONS

Calories Per Serving: 250 calories

Protein: 10 grams.

Fat: 10 grams.

Carbohydrates: 35 grams.

Cottage Cheese Pancakes

 2 SERVINGS
4 PANCAKES

 PREP TIME:
5 MIN

 COOK TIME:
10 MIN

INGREDIENTS

- 1 cup cottage cheese
- 2 large eggs
- 1/4 cup almond flour
- 1/4 teaspoon baking powder
- 1/2 teaspoon vanilla extract
- Cooking spray or butter for greasing the skillet
- Optional toppings: fresh berries, Greek yogurt, maple syrup

DIRECTIONS

1. Blend cottage cheese, eggs, almond flour, baking powder, and vanilla extract until smooth.
2. Warm a non-stick skillet over medium heat, then apply cooking spray or butter to prevent sticking.
3. Transfer the pancake batter onto the skillet to make pancakes.
4. Cook until bubbles begin to appear on the surface. When this happens, flip them and continue cooking until they turn golden brown.
5. Repeat with the remaining batter.
6. Serve hot with desired toppings.

NUTRITIONS
Calories Per Serving: 200 calories
Protein: 17 grams.
Fat: 14 grams.
Carbohydrates: 13 grams.

Veggie Breakfast Burrito

 1 BURRITO | PREP TIME: 10 MIN | COOK TIME: 10 MIN

INGREDIENTS

- 1 whole-grain or low-carb tortilla
- 2 large eggs, scrambled
- 1/4 cup black beans, drained and rinsed
- 1/4 cup diced bell peppers
- 1/4 cup diced onions
- 2 tablespoons shredded cheddar cheese
- 1 tablespoon salsa
- Salt and pepper to taste
- Cooking spray or olive oil for greasing the skillet

DIRECTIONS

1. Warm a non-stick skillet on medium heat and coat it with cooking spray or olive oil.
2. Sauté diced bell peppers and onions until tender.
3. Place the scrambled eggs in the skillet. Cook until they firm up.
4. Warm black beans.
5. Layer scrambled eggs, sautéed bell peppers and onions, black beans, shredded cheddar cheese, and salsa in the center of the tortilla.
6. Fold the edges of the tortilla over the filling, and then roll it up firmly into a burrito.
7. Heat in the skillet for 1-2 minutes on each side until crispy.
8. Serve hot with additional salsa if desired.

NUTRITIONS

Calories Per Serving: 300 calories

Protein: 20 grams.

Fat: 20 grams.

Carbohydrates: 33 grams.

Spinach and Mushroom Crustless Quiche

 4 SERVINGS | PREP TIME: 10 MIN | COOK TIME: 20-35 MIN

INGREDIENTS

- 1 tablespoon olive oil
- 1 cup sliced mushrooms
- 2 cups fresh spinach leaves
- 1/2 cup diced onions
- 4 large eggs
- Salt and pepper to taste
- 1/2 cup milk or unsweetened almond milk
- 1/2 cup shredded cheddar cheese

NUTRITIONS

Calories Per Serving: 200 calories

Protein: 14 grams.

Fat: 15 grams.

Carbohydrates: 6 grams

DIRECTIONS

1. Preheating the oven to 350°F (175°C) and lightly sprinkle a pie dish or quiche pan with cooking spray.
2. Place a skillet over medium heat and add the olive oil. Add sliced mushrooms and diced onions, cooking until softened, about 5 minutes.
3. Add fresh spinach leaves to the skillet, cooking until wilted, about 2 minutes.
4. Beat the pepper, eggs, milk, and salt in a mixing bowl.
5. Stir in cooked mushrooms, spinach, onions, and shredded cheddar cheese.
6. Transfer the mixture to a pie dish you have prepared.
7. Bake for 25-30 minutes, until the quiche is set and the top is golden brown.
8. Allow the quiche to cool briefly before slicing and serving.

Apple Cinnamon Overnight Oat

 1 SERVING | PREP TIME: 5 MIN | COOK TIME: OVERNIGHT

INGREDIENTS

- 1/2 cup old-fashioned oats
- 1/2 cup unsweetened almond milk
- 1/4 cup Greek yogurt
- 1/2 small apple, diced
- 1 tablespoon maple syrup or honey
- 1/2 teaspoon ground cinnamon
- 1 tablespoon chopped nuts (such as walnuts or almonds)

DIRECTIONS

1. Combine oats, almond milk, Greek yogurt, diced apple, maple syrup or honey, and ground cinnamon in a mason jar or container.
2. Stir well to combine all ingredients.
3. Cover and refrigerate overnight.
4. In the morning, stir the oats and top with chopped nuts before serving.
5. Enjoy cold or heat in the microwave if desired.

NUTRITIONS

Calories Per Serving: 250 calories

Protein: 7 grams.

Fat: 7 grams.

Carbohydrates: 38 grams.

Chapter 5

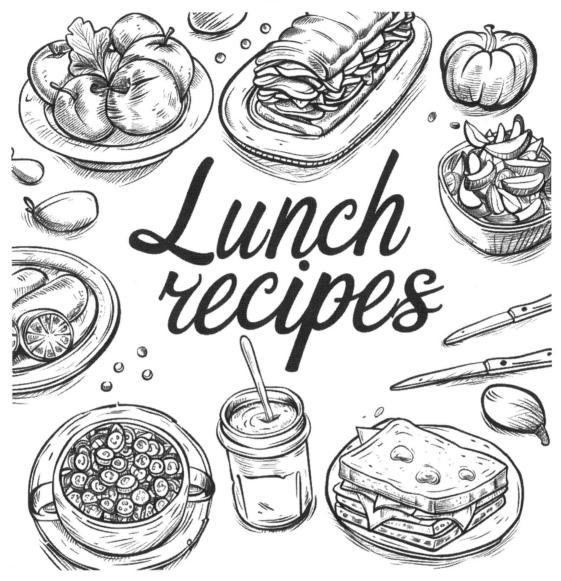

Introduction to Nutritious Midday Meals

Welcome to the Lunch Recipes chapter! This chapter will go through various flavorful and satisfying dishes perfect for lunch. These lunch recipes are suitable for individuals with diabetes mellitus (DM). They focus on incorporating lean proteins, healthy fats, fiber-rich vegetables, and complex carbohydrates with low glycemic index to help manage blood sugar levels. These recipes also emphasize portion control and the use of ingredients that contribute to overall health and well-being.

Tips for a Blood Sugar-Friendly Start to the Day:

Choose Low-Glycemic Foods: Opt for foods with a low glycemic index (GI), such as whole grains, non-starchy vegetables, and lean proteins. These foods are digested more slowly, leading to a gradual rise in blood sugar levels.

Include Protein: Protein helps stabilize blood sugar levels and keeps you feeling full longer. Add protein-rich foods like eggs, Greek yogurt, nuts, and seeds to your breakfast.

Add Fiber: Fiber-rich foods, such as fruits, vegetables, whole grains, and nuts, can help regulate blood sugar levels and improve digestion. Aim to include fiber in your breakfast to promote overall health.

Limit Added Sugars: Be mindful of added sugars in breakfast cereals, pastries, and sweetened beverages. Opt for unsweetened options or use natural sweeteners like honey or maple syrup in moderation.

Balance Carbohydrates: While carbohydrates are an important energy source, it's essential to balance them with protein and healthy fats to prevent blood sugar spikes. Choose complex carbohydrates like whole grains and limit refined carbs like white bread and sugary cereals.

Watch Portion Sizes: Pay attention to portion sizes to avoid overeating, which can lead to spikes in blood sugar levels. Use measuring cups and spoons to portion out foods like cereal, yogurt, and nuts.

Stay Hydrated: Drink plenty of water throughout the day, including breakfast. Staying hydrated helps maintain blood sugar levels and supports overall health.

Mindful Eating: Take your time to enjoy your breakfast and listen to your body's hunger and fullness cues. Eating mindfully can help prevent overeating and promote better blood sugar control.

Caprese Salad

 1 SALAD | PREP TIME: 5 MIN | COOK TIME: 5 MIN

INGREDIENTS

- 1 medium tomato, sliced
- 2 oz fresh mozzarella cheese, sliced
- 1 tablespoon balsamic glaze
- Fresh basil leaves
- Salt and pepper to taste

DIRECTIONS

1. Arrange tomato slices and fresh mozzarella cheese slices on a plate.
2. Drizzle balsamic glaze over the tomato and mozzarella.
3. Garnish with fresh basil leaves.
4. Season with salt and pepper to taste.
5. Serve immediately.

NUTRITIONS

Calories Per Serving: 200 calories

Protein: 12 grams per serving.

Fat: 14 grams per serving.

Carbohydrates: 9 grams per serving.

Veggie and Bean Quesadilla

 1 QUESADILLA | PREP TIME: 10 MIN | COOK TIME: 5-6 MIN

INGREDIENTS

- 2 whole grain or low-carb tortillas
- 1/4 cup black beans, drained and rinsed
- 1/4 cup diced bell peppers
- 1/4 cup diced onions
- 1/4 cup shredded cheddar cheese
- Cooking spray

NUTRITIONS

Calories Per Serving: 300 calories

Protein: 15 grams per quesadilla.

Fat: 10 grams per quesadilla.

Carbohydrates: 35 grams per quesadilla.

DIRECTIONS

1. To prepare a delicious quesadilla, follow these simple steps:
2. Begin by heating a non-stick skillet over medium heat. Lightly spray the skillet with cooking spray.
3. Once the skillet is hot, place a tortilla and evenly sprinkle some shredded cheddar cheese.
4. Next, add a generous helping of black beans, followed by diced bell peppers and onions. The bell peppers add a sweet crunch, while the onions provide a savory flavor.
5. Sprinkle the remaining shredded cheddar cheese over the vegetables.
6. Place the second tortilla on top of the cheese to create a quesadilla. Use a spatula to press the quesadilla gently to ensure even cooking.
7. Cook the quesadilla until the cheese is melted and the tortillas are crispy, 2-3 minutes on each side. The aroma of the melted cheese will waft through the kitchen, making your mouth water.
8. Once the quesadilla is perfect, slice it into wedges and serve hot. The crispy tortillas will provide a satisfying crunch, while the melted cheese and vegetables will burst with flavor in your mouth.
9. Use a non-stick skillet and cooking spray to ensure the quesadilla doesn't stick to the pan

Chicken Caesar Salad

 1 SERVING | PREP TIME: 10 MIN | COOK TIME: 10 MIN

INGREDIENTS

- 4 oz grilled chicken breast, sliced
- 2 cups romaine lettuce, chopped
- 1/4 cup cherry tomatoes, halved
- 2 tablespoons grated Parmesan cheese
- 2 tablespoons Caesar dressing
- 1/4 cup croutons (optional)

NUTRITIONS

Calories Per Serving: 300 calories

Protein: 30 grams per serving.

Fat: 20 grams per serving.

Carbohydrates: 10 grams per serving.

DIRECTIONS

1. Mix the sliced grilled chicken breast, cherry tomatoes, and chopped romaine lettuce in a spacious bowl.
2. Evenly drizzle Caesar dressing on the salad, ensuring each ingredient is appropriately coated.
3. Sprinkle-grated Parmesan cheese and, if desired, croutons over the salad.
4. Serve promptly for optimal freshness.

5. Use a non-stick skillet and cooking spray to ensure the quesadilla doesn't stick to the pan.

Egg Salad Lettuce Wraps

 2 SERVINGS | PREP TIME: 10 MIN | COOK TIME: 10 MIN

INGREDIENTS

- 2 hard-boiled eggs, chopped
- 2 tablespoons Greek yogurt
- 1 tablespoon Dijon mustard
- 1/4 cup diced celery
- Salt and pepper to taste
- 4 large lettuce leaves (such as butter lettuce or romaine)

DIRECTIONS

1. Combine chopped hard-boiled eggs, Greek yogurt, Dijon mustard, diced celery, salt, and pepper in a bowl.
2. Mix well until all ingredients are combined.
3. Divide the egg salad mixture evenly among the lettuce leaves.
4. Roll up the lettuce leaves to form wraps.
5. Serve immediately.

NUTRITIONS

Calories Per Serving: 200 calories

Protein: 12 grams per serving.

Fat: 14 grams per serving.

Carbohydrates: 6 grams per serving.

Turkey and Veggie Skewers

 2 SERVINGS | PREP TIME: 10 MIN | COOK TIME: 8-10 MIN

INGREDIENTS

- 4 oz turkey breast, cut into chunks
- 1/2 cup cherry tomatoes
- 1/2 cup bell peppers, cut into chunks
- 1/2 cup zucchini, sliced
- 1/4 cup red onion, cut into chunks
- Wooden skewers, soaked in water for 30 minutes

DIRECTIONS

1. Thread turkey breast chunks, cherry tomatoes, bell peppers, zucchini slices, and red onion chunks onto the wooden skewers.
2. Put on the heat and reduce it to medium. Place a grill pan over the heat and allow to heat for a minute.
3. Put the skewers in and grill them for about 8-10 minutes, turning them occasionally or until the turkey is cooked to the extent you want and the vegetables are tender.
4. Serve hot.

NUTRITIONS

Calories Per Serving: 250 calories

Protein: 28 grams per serving.

Fat: 6 grams per serving.

Carbohydrates: 12 grams per serving.

Mediterranean Hummus Bowl

 1 SERVING | PREP TIME: 10 MIN | COOK TIME: 10 MIN

INGREDIENTS

- 1/2 cup cooked quinoa
- 1/4 cup hummus
- 1/4 cup cherry tomatoes, halved
- 1/4 cup diced cucumber
- 1/4 cup diced red onion
- 2 tablespoons chopped Kalamata olives
- 2 tablespoons crumbled feta cheese
- Fresh parsley for garnish

DIRECTIONS

1. In a bowl, layer cooked quinoa, hummus, cherry tomatoes, diced cucumber, diced red onion, chopped Kalamata olives, and crumbled feta cheese.
2. Garnish with fresh parsley.
3. Serve chilled or at room temperature.

NUTRITIONS
Calories Per Serving: 300 calories
Protein: 12 grams per serving.
Fat: 15 grams per serving.
Carbohydrates: 30 grams per serving.

Veggie and Bean Wrap

 1 WRAP | PREP TIME: 5 MIN | COOK TIME: 5 MIN

INGREDIENTS

- 1 whole-grain or low-carb tortilla
- 1/4 cup black beans, drained and rinsed
- 1/4 cup diced bell peppers
- 1/4 cup diced tomatoes
- 2 tablespoons shredded cheddar cheese
- 2 tablespoons salsa

DIRECTIONS

1. Spread the tortilla flat on a clean surface and cover it with black beans evenly.
2. Layer diced bell peppers, tomatoes, shredded cheddar cheese, and salsa on the beans.
3. Roll up the tortilla tightly to form a wrap.
4. Slice in half and serve.

NUTRITIONS

Calories Per Serving: 250 calories

Protein: 12 grams per wrap.

Fat: 8 grams per wrap.

Carbohydrates: 30 grams per wrap.

Greek Yogurt Chicken Salad

 1 SERVING | PREP TIME: 10 MIN | COOK TIME: 10 MIN

INGREDIENTS

- 4 oz cooked chicken breast, shredded
- 2 tablespoons Greek yogurt
- 1 tablespoon lemon juice
- 1/4 cup diced celery
- 1/4 cup diced apple
- 1/4 cup halved grapes
- Salt and pepper to taste
- Lettuce leaves for serving

DIRECTIONS

1. In a bowl, combine shredded chicken breast, Greek yogurt, lemon juice, diced celery, diced apple, halved grapes, salt, and pepper.
2. Mix well until all ingredients are combined.
3. Serve chicken salad over lettuce leaves.

NUTRITIONS

Calories Per Serving: 250 calories

Protein: 26 grams per serving.

Fat: 10 grams per serving.

Carbohydrates: 12 grams per serving

Turkey and Avocado Salad

 1 SERVING | PREP TIME: 10 MIN | COOK TIME: 10 MIN

INGREDIENTS

- 4 oz sliced turkey breast
- 1/2 avocado, diced
- 2 cups mixed salad greens
- 1/4 cup cherry tomatoes, halved
- 1/4 cup diced cucumber
- 2 tablespoons balsamic vinaigrette dressing

DIRECTIONS

1. Combine sliced turkey breast, diced avocado, mixed salad greens, cherry tomatoes, and diced cucumber in a large bowl.
2. Drizzle balsamic vinaigrette dressing over the salad.
3. Toss gently to coat.
4. Serve immediately.

NUTRITIONS

Calories Per Serving: 300 calories

Protein: 20 grams per serving.

Fat: 20 grams per serving.

Carbohydrates: 15 grams per serving.

Grilled Chicken Salad

 1 SERVING PREP TIME: 10 MIN COOK TIME: 10 MIN

INGREDIENTS

- 4 oz grilled chicken breast, sliced
- 2 cups mixed salad greens
- ½ cup cherry tomatoes, halved
- ¼ cup sliced cucumber
- ¼ cup sliced bell peppers
- 2 tablespoons balsamic vinaigrette dressing

DIRECTIONS

5. Combine mixed salad greens, cherry tomatoes, cucumber, and bell peppers in a large bowl.
6. Add sliced grilled chicken breast on top.
7. Drizzle with balsamic vinaigrette dressing.
8. Gently toss to coat.
9. Serve immediatelly.

NUTRITIONS

Calories Per Serving: 300 calories

Protein: 30 grams per serving.

Fat: 12 grams per serving.

Carbohydrates: 15 grams per serving.

Vegetable and Lentil Soup

 2 SERVINGS | PREP TIME: 10 MIN | COOK TIME: 20 MIN

INGREDIENTS

- 1/2 cup cooked lentils
- 1 cup diced mixed vegetables (such as carrots, celery, onions, and potatoes)
- 2 cups low-sodium vegetable broth
- 1/2 teaspoon dried thyme
- 1/2 teaspoon dried rosemary
- Salt and pepper to taste
- Potential toppings: grated chopped fresh parsley, Parmesan cheese

DIRECTIONS

1. In a pot, combine cooked lentils, diced mixed vegetables, low-sodium vegetable broth, dried thyme, and dried rosemary.
2. Once all the ingredients are in, bring the mixture to a boil. After boiling, reduce the heat and let it simmer for 15-20 minutes or until the vegetables are tender.
3. Add salt and pepper to taste.
4. Once the soup is prepared, carefully ladle it into bowls. Garnish each bowl with chopped fresh parsley and grated Parmesan cheese according to your preference.
5. Serve hot.

NUTRITIONS

Calories Per Serving: 200 calories

Protein: 10 grams per serving.

Fat: 1 gram per serving.

Carbohydrates: 30 grams per serving.

Turkey and Avocado Wrap

 1 WRAP | PREP TIME: 5 MIN | COOK TIME: 5 MIN

INGREDIENTS

- 1 whole-grain or low-carb tortilla
- 3 oz sliced turkey breast
- 1/4 avocado, sliced
- 1/4 cup shredded lettuce
- 2 slices tomato
- 1 tablespoon hummus or mustard (optional)

DIRECTIONS

1. Lay the tortilla flat on a clean surface.
2. Spread hummus or mustard (if using) evenly over the tortilla.
3. On top, layer sliced turkey breast, avocado, shredded lettuce, and tomato slices.
4. Roll up the tortilla tightly to form a wrap.
5. Slice in half and serve.

NUTRITIONS

Calories Per Serving: 250 calories

Protein: 20 grams per wrap.

Fat: 10 grams per wrap.

Carbohydrates: 25 grams per wrap.

Quinoa and Vegetable Stir-Fry

 1 SERVING | PREP TIME: 10 MIN | COOK TIME: 10 MIN

INGREDIENTS

- 1/2 cup cooked quinoa
- 1 cup mixed vegetables (such as bell peppers, broccoli, carrots, and snap peas)
- 2 tablespoons low-sodium soy sauce
- 1 tablespoon sesame oil
- 1 teaspoon minced garlic
- 1 teaspoon minced ginger
- Optional toppings: sliced green onions, sesame seeds

NUTRITIONS

Calories Per Serving: 300 calories
Protein: 10 grams per serving.
Fat: 5 grams per serving.
Carbohydrates: 35 grams per serving.

DIRECTIONS

1. Begin by heating a skillet over medium heat. Once the skillet has heated, pour in some sesame oil.
2. Once the oil has heated up, add some minced garlic and ginger to the skillet.
3. Cook the garlic and ginger until they start to emit a fragrant aroma.
4. Once the aroma fills the air, toss some mixed vegetables into the skillet and stir-fry until they become tender-crisp.
5. Then, add some cooked quinoa and low-sodium soy sauce to the skillet and stir the ingredients together.
6. Cook them for 2-3 minutes, stirring occasionally to cook the ingredients evenly.
7. After everything is cooked, you can remove the skillet from the heat. If you want, you can garnish it with some slices of green onions and sesame.
8. Serve the dish hot and enjoy!

Tuna Salad Stuffed with Bell Peppers

 2 SERVINGS | PREP TIME: 10 MIN | COOK TIME: 10 MIN

INGREDIENTS

- 1 can (5 oz) tuna, drained
- 1/4 cup diced celery
- 1/4 cup diced red onion
- 2 tablespoons Greek yogurt
- 1 tablespoon lemon juice
- 1 teaspoon Dijon mustard
- 2 bell peppers, halved and seeds removed
- Salt and pepper to taste
- Parmesan cheese

DIRECTIONS

1. Combine drained tuna, diced celery, red onion, Greek yogurt, lemon juice, mustard, salt, and pepper in a bowl.
2. Mix well until all ingredients are combined.
3. Spoon the tuna salad mixture into the halved bell peppers, distributing evenly.
4. Serve immediately.

NUTRITIONS
Calories Per Serving: 200 calories

Protein: 15 grams per serving.

Fat: 5 grams per serving.

Carbohydrates: 10 grams per serving.

Veggie and Hummus Wrap

 1 SERVING | PREP TIME: 10 MIN | COOK TIME: 10 MIN

INGREDIENTS

- 1 whole-grain or low-carb tortilla
- 2 tablespoons hummus
- 1/4 cup shredded carrots
- 1/4 cup sliced cucumbers
- 1/4 cup sliced bell peppers
- 1/4 cup baby spinach leaves

DIRECTIONS

1. Spread hummus evenly over the tortilla.
2. Arrange shredded carrots, sliced cucumbers, bell peppers, and baby spinach leaves in layers atop the hummus.
3. Carefully roll the tortilla to create a tightly wrapped wrap.
4. Slice in half and serve.

NUTRITIONS

Calories Per Serving: 200 calories

Protein: 5 grams per wrap.

Fat: 10 grams per wrap.

Carbohydrates: 25 grams per wrap.

Turkey and Vegetable Stir-Fry

 2 SERVINGS | PREP TIME: 10 MIN | COOK TIME: 10 MIN

INGREDIENTS

- 4 oz sliced turkey breast
- 1 cup mixed vegetables (such as bell peppers, broccoli, carrots, and snap peas)
- 1 tablespoon low-sodium soy sauce
- 1 tablespoon olive oil
- 1/2 teaspoon minced garlic
- Salt and pepper to taste

DIRECTIONS

1. Heat some olive oil in a skillet over medium heat.
2. Throw some minced garlic into the skillet and cook until the aroma is released.
3. Add sliced turkey breast to the skillet and cook until it turns brown.
4. Add several different mixes of vegetables into the skillet and stir-fry until they are tender-crisp.
5. Mix in some low-sodium soy sauce and cook for 2-3 minutes.
6. Add some salt and pepper to taste.
7. Serve it hot.

NUTRITIONS

Calories Per Serving: 250 calories

Protein: 20 grams per serving.

Fat: 10 grams per serving.

Carbohydrates: 15 grams per serving.

Mediterranean Chickpea Salad

 2 SERVINGS | PREP TIME: 10 MIN | COOK TIME: 10 MIN

INGREDIENTS

- 1 cup cooked chickpeas
- 1/4 cup diced cucumber
- 1/4 cup diced tomatoes
- 1/4 cup diced red onion
- 2 tablespoons chopped fresh parsley
- 1 tablespoon olive oil
- 1 tablespoon lemon juice
- Salt and pepper to taste
- Optional toppings: crumbled feta cheese, sliced olives

DIRECTIONS

1. Combine cooked chickpeas, diced cucumber, tomatoes, red onion, and chopped fresh parsley in a bowl.
2. Sprinkle lemon juice and olive oil on the salad, ensure it is evenly covered, and salt and pepper, depending on your taste.
3. Toss gently to coat.
4. Garnish with crumbled feta cheese and sliced olives if desired.
5. Serve chilled or at room temperature.

NUTRITIONS

Calories Per Serving: 200 calories

Protein: 10 grams per serving.

Fat: 5 grams per serving.

Carbohydrates: 25 grams per serving.

Chapter 6

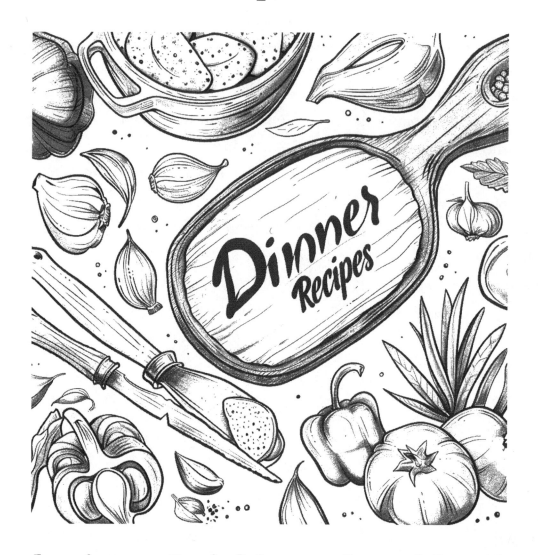

Introduction to Satisfying and Healthy Dinners

This chapter is about delicious dinner recipes —tasty and diabetes-friendly dishes perfect for any evening meal. Within these pages, you'll find flavorful recipes designed to make dinnertime enjoyable and nutritious. Each recipe has detailed instructions and helpful tips for a stress-free cooking experience.

Baked Lemon Herb Salmon

 1 SERVING | PREP TIME: 5 MIN | COOK TIME: 12-15 MIN

INGREDIENTS

- 4 oz salmon fillet
- 1 tablespoon olive oil
- 1 tablespoon fresh lemon juice
- 1 teaspoon minced garlic
- 1 teaspoon chopped fresh parsley
- Salt and pepper to taste

DIRECTIONS

1. Preheat oven to 375°F (190°C).
2. Whisk together olive oil, lemon juice, pepper, minced garlic, chopped parsley, and salt in a small bowl.
3. Line a baking sheet with parchment paper, and arrange the salmon fillet.
4. Evenly pour the lemon herb mixture over the salmon.
5. Place in the oven and leave for about 12-15 minutes until you are sure the salmon is thoroughly cooked and flakes easily with a fork.
6. Serve the salmon hot.

NUTRITIONS

Calories Per Serving: 300 calories

Protein: 25 grams per serving

Fat: 20 grams per serving

Carbohydrates: 3 grams per serving

Vegetable and Chickpea Stir-Fry

 1 SERVING | PREP TIME: 10 MIN | COOK TIME: 10 MIN

INGREDIENTS

- 1/2 cup cooked chickpeas
- 1 cup mixed vegetables (such as bell peppers, broccoli, carrots, and snap peas)
- 2 tablespoons low-sodium soy sauce
- 1 tablespoon sesame oil
- 1 teaspoon minced garlic
- 1 teaspoon minced ginger
- Optional toppings: sliced green onions, sesame seeds

NUTRITIONS

Calories Per Serving: 300 calories

Protein: 10 grams per serving

Fat: 10 grams per serving

Carbohydrates: 25 grams per serving

DIRECTIONS

1. Turn the heat to medium, place the skillet on, and add some garlic and ginger until aromatic.
2. Put the mixed vegetables into the skillet on the heat and stir-fry until they reach a tender-crisp texture.
3. Add the mixed vegetables to the skillet on the heat and stir-fry until they reach a tender-crisp texture.
4. Incorporate the cooked chickpeas and low-sodium soy sauce into the skillet.
5. Continue cooking for an extra 2-3 minutes, occasionally stirring.
6. Once done, remove it from the heat.
7. Add sesame seeds and sliced green onion to garnish.
8. Serve hot.

Turkey and Vegetable Skillet

 1 SERVING | PREP TIME: 10 MIN | COOK TIME: 15 MIN

INGREDIENTS

- 4 oz ground turkey
- 1 cup mixed vegetables (such as bell peppers, onions, zucchini, and tomatoes)
- 1 tablespoon olive oil
- 1 teaspoon minced garlic
- 1/2 teaspoon dried oregano
- Salt and pepper to taste

DIRECTIONS

1. Warm olive oil in a skillet over medium heat.
2. Introduce minced garlic to the skillet and cook until it becomes fragrant.
3. Incorporate ground turkey into the skillet and cook until it browns.
4. Add mixed vegetables to the skillet and sauté until they become tender.
5. Season with dried oregano, salt, and pepper according to your preference.
6. Continue cooking for an additional 2-3 minutes, stirring occasionally.
7. Serve while hot.

NUTRITIONS

Calories Per Serving: 250 calories

Protein: 20 grams per serving

Fat: 10 grams per serving

Carbohydrates: 10 grams per serving

Cauliflower Fried Rice

 1 SERVING | PREP TIME: 10 MIN | COOK TIME: 10 MIN

INGREDIENTS

- 1 cup cauliflower rice
- 1/4 cup diced mixed vegetables (such as carrots, peas, and bell peppers)
- 2 tablespoons low-sodium soy sauce
- 1 tablespoon sesame oil
- 1 teaspoon minced garlic
- 1 teaspoon minced ginger
- 1 egg, beaten
- Optional toppings: sliced green onions, sesame seeds

NUTRITIONS

Calories Per Serving: 200 calories

Protein: 5 grams per serving

Fat: 15 grams per serving

Carbohydrates: 15 grams per serving

DIRECTIONS

1. Heat sesame oil in a skillet over medium heat.
2. Add minced garlic and ginger to the skillet and cook until fragrant.
3. Add diced mixed vegetables to the skillet and sauté until tender.
4. Stir in cauliflower rice and low-sodium soy sauce.
5. Move the cauliflower rice mixture to a side of the skillet and add the beaten egg to the other side.
6. Scramble the egg until cooked, then mix it into the cauliflower rice mixture.
7. Continue cooking for another 2-3 minutes, occasionally stirring.
8. Then, remove the heat and garnish with sliced green onions and sesame seeds.
9. Serve hot.

Lemon Garlic Shrimp Pasta

 1 SERVING | PREP TIME: 10 MIN | COOK TIME: 10 MIN

INGREDIENTS

- 2 oz whole grain or low-carb pasta
- 4 oz shrimp, peeled and deveined
- 1 tablespoon olive oil
- 1 teaspoon minced garlic
- 1 tablespoon fresh lemon juice
- 1 tablespoon chopped fresh parsley
- Salt and pepper to taste

DIRECTIONS

1. Cook pasta according to package instructions. Drain and set aside.
2. Heat olive oil in a skillet over medium heat.
3. Once heated, add diced garlic to the skillet and cook until it becomes fragrant.
4. Next, put the shrimp in the skillet and cook until it turns pink and opaque.
5. Then, stir the pasta with fresh lemon juice, chopped parsley, salt, and pepper.
6. Continue cooking while stirring from time to time or for an additional 2-3 minutes, occasionally stirring.

NUTRITIONS

Calories Per Serving: 300 calories

Protein: 20 grams per serving

Fat: 10 grams per serving

Carbohydrates: 25 grams per serving

Baked Chicken and Vegetable Casserole

 1 SERVING | PREP TIME: 10 MIN | COOK TIME: 20-25 MIN

INGREDIENTS

- 4 oz chicken breast, diced
- 1 cup mixed vegetables (such as broccoli, cauliflower, carrots, and bell peppers)
- 1 tablespoon olive oil
- 1 teaspoon minced garlic
- 1/2 teaspoon dried thyme
- Salt and pepper to taste
- Optional topping: shredded mozzarella cheese

DIRECTIONS

1. Preheat oven to 375°F (190°C).
2. Toss diced chicken breast and mixed vegetables with olive oil, minced garlic, dried thyme, salt, and pepper in a bowl.
3. Transfer the mixture of the chicken and vegetables into a baking dish.
4. Bake in the preheated oven for 20-25 minutes or until the vegetables appear tender and the chicken is well cooked.
5. If desired, sprinkle shredded mozzarella cheese over the casserole during the last 5 minutes of baking.
6. Serve hot.

NUTRITIONS

Calories Per Serving: 300 calories

Protein: 25 grams per serving

Fat: 15 grams per serving

Carbohydrates: 10 grams per serving

Beef and Broccoli Stir-Fry

 1 SERVING | PREP TIME: 20 MIN | COOK TIME: 8-10 MIN

INGREDIENTS

- 4 oz lean beef, thinly sliced
- 1 cup broccoli florets
- 1 tablespoon low-sodium soy sauce
- 1 teaspoon cornstarch
- 1 teaspoon minced garlic
- 1 teaspoon minced ginger
- 1/2 teaspoon sesame oil
- Salt and pepper to taste

DIRECTIONS

1. In a small bowl, whisk together low-sodium soy sauce, cornstarch, minced garlic, ginger, sesame oil, salt, and pepper.
2. Marinate sliced beef in the soy sauce mixture for 30 minutes in the refrigerator.
3. Heat a skillet or wok over medium-high heat.
4. Add the marinated beef and stir-fry until browned and cooked through.
5. Add broccoli florets to the skillet and stir-fry for 2-3 minutes or until tender-crisp.
6. Serve hot.

NUTRITIONS

Calories Per Serving: 250 calories

Protein: 25 grams per serving

Fat: 10 grams per serving

Carbohydrates: 10 grams per serving

Grilled Lemon Herb Chicken

 1 SERVING   PREP TIME: 35 MIN   COOK TIME: 12-16 MIN

INGREDIENTS

- 4 oz chicken breast
- 1 tablespoon olive oil
- 1 tablespoon fresh lemon juice
- 1 teaspoon minced garlic
- 1 teaspoon chopped fresh rosemary
- Salt and pepper to taste

NUTRITIONS

Calories Per Serving: 250 calories

Protein: 25 grams per serving

Fat: 15 grams per serving

Carbohydrates: 2 grams per serving

DIRECTIONS

1. Combine olive oil, lemon juice, minced garlic, chopped rosemary, salt, and pepper in a bowl, mixing them thoroughly.

2. Place the chicken breast in the marinade, ensuring it's evenly coated. Let it marinate in the refrigerator for at least 30 minutes.

3. Preheat the grill to medium-high heat.

4. Remove the chicken breast from the marinade and grill each side for 6-8 minutes or until fully cooked. Serve immediately while hot.

Veggie and Tofu Stir-Fry

 1 SERVING | PREP TIME: 10 MIN | COOK TIME: 10 MIN

INGREDIENTS

- 4 oz firm tofu, cubed
- 1 cup mixed vegetables (such as bell peppers, mushrooms, snap peas, and carrots)
- 2 tablespoons low-sodium soy sauce
- 1 tablespoon sesame oil
- 1 teaspoon minced garlic
- 1 teaspoon minced ginger
- Salt and pepper to taste

DIRECTIONS

1. Warm sesame oil in a skillet over medium heat.
2. Introduce minced garlic and ginger to the skillet, cooking until their aroma emerges.
3. Incorporate cubed tofu into the skillet, cooking until it achieves a light brown hue.
4. Add mixed vegetables into the skillet and stir-fry until they reach a tender-crisp texture.
5. Stir in low-sodium soy sauce and cook for 2-3 minutes.
6. Season with salt and pepper to taste.
7. Serve hot.

NUTRITIONS

Calories Per Serving: 200 calories

Protein: 12 grams per serving

Fat: 14 grams per serving

Carbohydrates: 15 grams per serving

Zucchini Noodles with Marinara Sauce

 1 SERVING

 PREP TIME: 10 MIN

 COOK TIME: 10 MIN

INGREDIENTS

- 1 medium zucchini
- 1/2 cup marinara sauce (store-bought or homemade)
- 1 tablespoon olive oil
- 1 teaspoon minced garlic
- Salt and pepper to taste
- Optional toppings: grated Parmesan cheese, chopped fresh basil

DIRECTIONS

1. Spiralize the zucchini into noodles with a spiralizer. Heat olive oil in a skillet over medium heat, add the minced garlic, and cook until fragrant.
2. Add zucchini noodles to the skillet and sauté for 2-3 minutes or until tender.
3. Pour marinara sauce over the zucchini noodles and toss to coat.
4. Cook for an additional 2-4 minutes, stirring occasionally.
5. Season with salt and pepper to taste.
6. Serve hot with optional toppings if desired.

NUTRITIONS

Calories Per Serving: 150 calories
Protein: 3 grams per serving
Fat: 7 grams per serving
Carbohydrates: 10 grams per serving

Quinoa Stuffed Bell Peppers

 1 SERVING | PREP TIME: 15 MIN | COOK TIME: 25-30 MIN

INGREDIENTS

- 2 bell peppers, halved and seeds removed
- 1/2 cup cooked quinoa
- 1/4 cup black beans, drained and rinsed
- 1/4 cup diced tomatoes
- 1/4 cup diced red onion
- 1/4 cup corn kernels (fresh or frozen)
- 1/4 teaspoon cumin
- Salt and pepper to taste
- Optional toppings: shredded cheddar cheese, chopped fresh cilantro

DIRECTIONS

1. Preheat oven to 375°F (190°C).
2. Combine or mix the cooked quinoa, black beans, tomatoes, red onion, corn kernels, cumin, salt, and pepper in a bowl.
3. Spoon the quinoa mixture into the halved bell peppers, dividing evenly.
4. Put the stuffed bell peppers onto a baking sheet lined with parchment paper.
5. Cover the baking sheet with aluminum foil and bake for 30-35 minutes or until the bell peppers appear tender.
6. Sprinkle shredded cheddar cheese over the stuffed bell peppers during the last 5 minutes of baking.
7. Serve hot with optional toppings if desired.

NUTRITIONS

Calories Per Serving: 200 calories

Protein: 7 grams per serving

Fat: 2 grams per serving

Carbohydrates: 35 grams per serving

Eggplant Parmesant

 2 SERVINGS

 PREP TIME: 10 MIN

 COOK TIME: 25-35 MIN

INGREDIENTS

- 1 small eggplant, sliced into rounds
- 1/2 cup marinara sauce (store-bought or homemade)
- 1/4 cup shredded mozzarella cheese
- 2 tablespoons grated Parmesan cheese
- 1 tablespoon olive oil
- 1/4 teaspoon dried oregano
- Salt and pepper to taste

DIRECTIONS

1. Preheat oven to 375°F (190°C).
2. Brush both sides of the slices of eggplant with olive oil and season with dried oregano, salt, and pepper.
3. Put the slices of eggplant on a baking sheet lined with parchment paper.
4. Bake for 15-20 minutes or until the eggplant is tender.
5. Remove from oven and place marinara sauce, shredded mozzarella cheese, and grated Parmesan cheese on each slice of eggplant.
6. Return to the oven and bake for 10-15 minutes or until the cheese is melted and bubbly.
7. Serve hot.

NUTRITIONS

Calories Per Serving: 200 calories

Protein: 7 grams per serving

Fat: 10 grams per serving

Carbohydrates: 15 grams per serving

Baked Stuffed Bell Peppers

 2 SERVINGS | PREP TIME: 15 MIN | COOK TIME: 25-30 MIN

INGREDIENTS

- 2 bell peppers, halved and seeds removed
- 1/2 cup cooked quinoa
- 1/4 cup black beans, drained and rinsed
- 1/4 cup diced tomatoes
- 1/4 cup diced red onion
- 1/4 cup corn kernels (fresh or frozen)
- 1/4 teaspoon cumin
- Salt and pepper to taste
- Optional toppings: shredded cheddar cheese, chopped fresh cilantro

DIRECTIONS

1. Preheat oven to 375°F (190°C).
2. In a bowl, combine cooked quinoa, black beans, diced tomatoes, diced red onion, corn kernels, cumin, salt, and pepper.
3. Spoon the quinoa mixture into the halved bell peppers, dividing evenly.
4. Place the stuffed bell peppers on a baking sheet lined with parchment paper.
5. Cover the baking sheet with aluminum foil and bake for 25-30 minutes or until the bell peppers are tender.
6. Sprinkle shredded cheddar cheese over the stuffed bell peppers during the last 5 minutes of baking.
7. Serve hot with optional toppings if desired.

NUTRITIONS
Calories Per Serving: 200 calories
Protein: 9 grams per serving

Fat: 1 gram per serving

Carbohydrates: 25 grams per serving

Turkey Taco Lettuce Wraps

 2 SERVINGS | PREP TIME: 10 MIN | COOK TIME: 10 MIN

INGREDIENTS

- 4 oz ground turkey
- 1/4 cup diced onion
- 1/4 cup diced bell peppers
- 2 tablespoons taco seasoning
- 4 large lettuce leaves (such as butter lettuce or romaine)
- Optional toppings: diced tomatoes, shredded cheddar cheese, salsa, avocado slices

DIRECTIONS

1. In a skillet over medium heat, cook ground turkey until browned.
2. Add diced onion and bell peppers to the skillet and cook until softened.
3. Stir in taco seasoning and cook for an additional 2-3 minutes.
4. Spoon the turkey mixture onto lettuce leaves.
5. Top with optional toppings if desired.
6. Serve immediately.

NUTRITIONS

Calories Per Serving: 200 calories
Protein: 15 grams per serving
Fat: 5 grams per serving
Carbohydrates: 10 grams per serving

Lemon Garlic Shrimp Skewers

 2 SERVINGS | PREP TIME: 40 MIN | COOK TIME: 6-8 MIN

INGREDIENTS

- 8 oz shrimp, peeled and deveined
- 2 cloves garlic, minced
- 2 tablespoons olive oil
- 1 tablespoon fresh lemon juice
- 1 teaspoon lemon zest
- 1 teaspoon chopped fresh parsley
- Salt and pepper to taste

DIRECTIONS

1. Combine minced garlic, olive oil, lemon juice, lemon zest, chopped parsley, salt, and pepper in a bowl.
2. Add shrimp to the bowl and toss to coat evenly.
3. Cover and refrigerate for 30 minutes to marinate.
4. Preheat the grill to medium-high heat.
5. Thread marinated shrimp onto skewers.
6. Grill shrimp skewers for 2-3 minutes per side or until shrimp are pink and opaque.
7. Serve hot.

NUTRITIONS

Calories Per Serving: 200 calories

Protein: 20 grams per serving

Fat: 10 grams per serving

Carbohydrates: 4 grams per serving

Spinach and Feta Stuffed Chicken Breast

 1 SERVING | PREP TIME: 15 MIN | COOK TIME: 25-30 MIN

INGREDIENTS

- 4 oz chicken breast
- 1 cup fresh spinach leaves
- 1 tablespoon crumbled feta cheese
- 1 teaspoon olive oil
- 1/2 teaspoon minced garlic
- Salt and pepper to taste

NUTRITIONS

Calories Per Serving: 250 calories

Protein: 25 grams per serving

Fat: 10 grams per serving

Carbohydrates: 2 grams per serving

DIRECTIONS

1. Preheat oven to 375°F (190°C).
2. Butterfly the chicken breast by slicing it horizontally, leaving one edge intact, and opening it like a book.
3. Season the inside of the chicken breast with salt and pepper.
4. Layer spinach leaves and crumbled feta cheese on one side of the chicken breast.
5. Fold the other side of the chicken breast over the filling to enclose it.
6. In a small bowl, combine olive oil and minced garlic.
7. Brush the outside of the stuffed chicken breast with the garlic-infused olive oil.
8. Place the stuffed chicken breast on a baking sheet lined with parchment paper.
9. Bake for 25-30 minutes or until the chicken is cooked through.
10. Serve hot.

Turkey and Quinoa Stuffed Peppers

 2 SERVINGS | PREP TIME: 20 MIN | COOK TIME: 25-30 MIN

INGREDIENTS

- 2 bell peppers, halved and seeds removed
- 1/2 cup cooked quinoa
- 4 oz lean ground turkey
- 1/4 cup diced tomatoes
- 1/4 cup diced onion
- 1/4 cup black beans, drained and rinsed
- 1/2 teaspoon chili powder
- Salt and pepper to taste
- Optional toppings: shredded cheddar cheese, chopped fresh cilantro

NUTRITIONS

Calories Per Serving: 250 calories

Protein: 15 grams per serving
Fat: 5 grams per serving
Carbohydrates: 20 grams per serving

DIRECTIONS

1. Preheat oven to 375°F (190°C).
2. In a skillet over medium heat, cook ground turkey until browned.
3. Add diced onion to the skillet and cook until softened.
4. Stir in diced tomatoes, black beans, cooked quinoa, chili powder, salt, and pepper. Cook for an additional 2-3 minutes.
5. Spoon the turkey and quinoa mixture into the halved bell peppers, dividing evenly.
6. Place the stuffed bell peppers on a baking sheet lined with parchment paper.
7. Cover the baking sheet with aluminum foil and bake for 25-30 minutes or until the bell peppers are tender.
8. Sprinkle shredded cheddar cheese over the stuffed bell peppers during the last 5 minutes of baking.
9. Serve hot with optional toppings if desired.

Balsamic Glazed Salmon

 1 SERVING | PREP TIME: 20 MIN | COOK TIME: 8-10 MIN

INGREDIENTS

- 4 oz salmon fillet
- 1 tablespoon balsamic vinegar
- 1 teaspoon honey
- 1/2 teaspoon minced garlic
- Salt and pepper to taste
- Optional garnish: chopped fresh parsley

DIRECTIONS

1. Whisk together balsamic vinegar, honey, minced garlic, salt, and pepper in a small bowl.
2. Place the salmon fillet in a shallow dish and pour the balsamic mixture over it. Let it marinate for 15-20 minutes.
3. Preheat the grill to medium-high heat.
4. Remove the salmon fillet from the marinade and discard the marinade.
5. Grill the salmon for 4-5 minutes per side or until cooked through and flaky.
6. Serve hot with optional garnish if desired.

NUTRITIONS

Calories Per Serving: 250 calories

Protein: 20 grams per serving

Fat: 10 grams per serving

Carbohydrates: 4 grams per serving

Turkey and Vegetable Meatballs

 2 SERVINGS | PREP TIME: 15 MIN | COOK TIME: 20-15 MIN

INGREDIENTS

- 4 oz lean ground turkey
- 1/4 cup grated zucchini
- 1/4 cup grated carrot
- 1/4 cup diced onion
- 1/4 cup whole wheat breadcrumbs
- 1 egg
- 1 teaspoon Italian seasoning
- Salt and pepper to taste
- Cooking spray

DIRECTIONS

1. Preheat oven to 375°F (190°C). Line a baking sheet with parchment paper and lightly coat it with cooking spray.

2. Combine ground turkey, grated zucchini, carrot, diced onion, breadcrumbs, egg, Italian seasoning, salt, and pepper in a large bowl. Mix until well combined.

3. Shape the mixture into meatballs about 1 inch in diameter and place them on the prepared baking sheet.

4. Bake for 20-25 minutes or until the meatballs are cooked and browned outside.

5. Serve hot with your favorite marinara sauce or as desired.

NUTRITIONS
Calories Per Serving: 200 calories
Protein: 20 grams per serving
Fat: 8 grams per serving
Carbohydrates: 15 grams per serving

Asian-Inspired Beef Lettuce Wraps

 2 SERVINGS | PREP TIME: 10 MIN | COOK TIME: 10 MIN

INGREDIENTS

- 4 oz lean ground beef
- 2 tablespoons hoisin sauce
- 1 tablespoon low-sodium soy sauce
- 1 teaspoon sesame oil
- 1 teaspoon minced garlic
- 1 teaspoon minced ginger
- 1/4 cup diced bell peppers
- 1/4 cup shredded carrots
- 4 large lettuce leaves (such as butter lettuce or romaine)
- Optional toppings: sliced green onions, chopped peanuts

NUTRITIONS

Calories Per Serving: 250 calories

Protein: 15 grams per serving

Fat: 10 grams per serving

Carbohydrates: 10 grams per serving

DIRECTIONS

1. In a skillet over medium heat, cook ground beef until browned.
2. Add minced garlic and minced ginger to the skillet and cook until fragrant.
3. Stir in hoisin sauce, low-sodium soy sauce, and sesame oil until well combined.
4. Add diced bell peppers and shredded carrots to the skillet and cook until softened.
5. Spoon the beef mixture onto lettuce leaves.
6. Top with optional toppings if desired.
7. Serve immediately.

Chapter 7

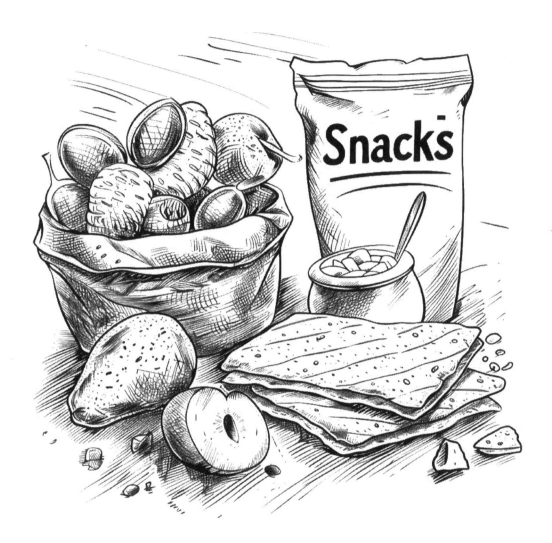

Snacks

Snacking can be essential to managing diabetes, helping to keep blood sugar levels stable between meals. In this chapter, we'll explore seven delicious and diabetes-friendly snack recipes that are easy to prepare and packed with nutrients to satisfy you throughout the day.

Introduction to Smart Snacking

Snacking is crucial in managing diabetes effectively and maintaining stable blood sugar levels throughout the day. For individuals with diabetes, strategic snacking can help prevent blood sugar spikes and crashes, provide sustained energy, and avoid overeating at main meals. Incorporating balanced snacks into your daily routine supports your overall health and well-being while enjoying delicious and satisfying treats.

The snack recipes in this chapter are specifically tailored to meet the unique nutritional needs of individuals with diabetes. Each recipe is carefully crafted to include a balance of carbohydrates, protein, and healthy fats, making them ideal for supporting blood sugar control and promoting satiety between meals. Whether craving something sweet, savory, or crunchy, you'll find various options to suit your taste preferences and dietary requirements.

One of the challenges of managing diabetes is ensuring you always have healthy snack options, especially when hunger strikes between meals or during busy days. That's where the snack recipes in this chapter come in handy. By preparing these snacks in advance and keeping them readily available, you can avoid reaching for less healthy options and ensure that you always have nutritious choices at your fingertips. From protein-packed energy balls to flavorful veggie dips and crunchy roasted chickpeas, these snacks are convenient and perfect for satisfying cravings while keeping blood sugar levels in check.

This chapter provides delicious snack ideas and valuable tips and strategies for making smart snacking choices throughout the day. From portion control and mindful eating to reading food labels and planning, you'll learn how to navigate snack time confidently and make choices supporting your health and wellness goals. By incorporating these tips into your daily routine, you can enjoy snacking without compromising your diabetes management plan.

Remember, snacking should be enjoyable and satisfying, not stressful or restrictive. With the proper knowledge and tools, you can make informed choices about your snacks and feel confident managing your diabetes effectively. So, explore the delicious snack recipes in this chapter and discover new ways to enjoy nutritious and flavorful treats while supporting your overall health and well-being.

Apple Slices with Peanut Butter

 1 SERVING | PREP TIME: 5 MIN | COOK TIME: 5 MIN

INGREDIENTS

- 1 medium apple, sliced
- 1 tablespoon natural peanut butter

DIRECTIONS

1. Spread peanut butter on apple slices.
2. Serve and enjoy!

NUTRITIONS

Calories Per Serving: 150 calories

Protein: 3 grams

Fat: 8 grams

Carbohydrates: 18 grams

Veggie Sticks with Hummus

 1 SERVING | PREP TIME: 5 MIN | COOK TIME: 5 MIN

INGREDIENTS

- 1 medium carrot, cut into sticks
- 1 medium cucumber, cut into sticks
- 2 tablespoons hummus

DIRECTIONS

1. Arrange carrot and cucumber sticks on a plate.
2. Serve with hummus for dipping.
3. Enjoy!

NUTRITIONS

Calories Per Serving: 100 calories

Protein: 3 grams

Fat: 6 grams

Carbohydrates: 9 grams

Cottage Cheese and Pineaple

 1 SERVING

 PREP TIME:
5 MIN

 COOK TIME:
5 MIN

INGREDIENTS

- 1/2 cup low-fat cottage cheese
- 1/2 cup diced pineapple (fresh or canned in juice)

DIRECTIONS

1. In a bowl, combine cottage cheese and diced pineapple.
2. Mix well and serve.

NUTRITIONS

Calories Per Serving: 150 calories

Protein: 14 grams

Fat: 1 gram

Carbohydrates: 20 grams

Hard-Boiles Eggs with Avocado

 1 SERVING | PREP TIME: 10 MIN | COOK TIME: 10 MIN

INGREDIENTS

- 2 hard-boiled eggs
- 1/2 avocado, sliced
- Salt and pepper to taste

DIRECTIONS

1. Peel the hard-boiled eggs and slice them in half.
2. Top each egg half with avocado slices.
3. Season with salt and pepper to taste.
4. Serve and enjoy!

NUTRITIONS

Calories Per Serving: 200 calories

Protein: 13 grams

Fat: 17 grams

Carbohydrates: 4 grams

Trail Mix

 1 SERVING | PREP TIME: 5 MIN | COOK TIME: 5 MIN

INGREDIENTS

- 1/4 cup mixed nuts (such as almonds, cashews, walnuts)
- 1/4 cup dried fruit (such as raisins or cranberries)
- 1 tablespoon dark chocolate chips (optional)

DIRECTIONS

1. Combine mixed nuts, dried fruit, and dark chocolate chips in a bowl.
2. Mix well and portion into individual servings.
3. Enjoy as a quick and satisfying snack.

NUTRITIONS

Calories Per Serving: 200 calories

Protein: 5 grams

Fat: 14 grams

Carbohydrates: 19 grams

Edamame

 1 SERVING | PREP TIME: 10 MIN | COOK TIME: 10 MIN

INGREDIENTS

- 1/2 cup cooked edamame (shelled soybeans)
- Salt to taste

DIRECTIONS

1. Steam or boil edamame according to package instructions.
2. Drain and sprinkle with salt while still warm.
3. Serve and enjoy!

NUTRITIONS

Calories Per Serving: 100 calories

Protein: 8 grams

Fat: 3 grams

Carbohydrates: 5 grams

Caprese Skewers

 1 SERVING | PREP TIME: 10 MIN | COOK TIME: 10 MIN

INGREDIENTS

- 6 cherry tomatoes
- 6 small fresh mozzarella balls
- 6 fresh basil leaves
- Balsamic glaze (optional)

DIRECTIONS

1. Thread a cherry tomato, a mozzarella ball, and a basil leaf onto a skewer.
2. Repeat with the remaining ingredients.
3. Drizzle with balsamic glaze if desired.
4. Serve immediately.

NUTRITIONS

Calories Per Serving: 100 calories

Protein: 7 grams

Fat: 5 grams

Carbohydrates: 4 grams

Simple Salad

 2 SERVINGS | PREP TIME: 10 MIN | COOK TIME: 10 MIN

INGREDIENTS

- 1 cucumber, diced
- 1 cup cherry tomatoes, halved
- 1/4 cup diced red onion
- 2 tablespoons chopped fresh parsley
- 1 tablespoon olive oil
- 1 tablespoon red wine vinegar
- Salt and pepper to taste

DIRECTIONS

1. red onion, and chopped parsley in a bowl.
2. Combine olive oil and red wine vinegar in a small bowl, whisking them together until well blended.
3. Drizzle the dressing over the salad and toss it gently to ensure all the ingredients are evenly coated.
4. Season with salt and pepper to taste.
5. Serve chilled.

NUTRITIONS

Calories Per Serving: 100 calories

Protein: 2 grams

Fat: 7 grams

Carbohydrates: 9 grams

Avocado Egg Salad

 1 SERVING | PREP TIME: 10 MIN | COOK TIME: 10 MIN

INGREDIENTS

- 2 hard-boiled eggs, chopped
- 1/2 avocado, mashed
- 1 tablespoon plain Greek yogurt
- 1 teaspoon Dijon mustard
- Salt and pepper to taste
- Optional: chopped chives for garnish

DIRECTIONS

1. Combine chopped hard-boiled eggs, mashed avocado, Greek yogurt, and Dijon mustard in a bowl.
2. Mix well until combined.
3. Season with salt and pepper to taste.
4. Garnish with chopped chives if desired.
5. Serve chilled.

NUTRITIONS

Calories Per Serving: 200 calories

Protein: 13 grams

Fat: 20 grams

Carbohydrates: 6 grams

Tuna Cucumber Bites

 1 SERVING | PREP TIME: 10 MIN | COOK TIME: 10 MIN

INGREDIENTS

- 1 small cucumber, sliced into rounds
- 1/4 cup canned tuna, drained
- 1 tablespoon plain Greek yogurt
- 1 teaspoon Dijon mustard
- Salt and pepper to taste

DIRECTIONS

1. Combine canned tuna, Greek yogurt, and Dijon mustard in a bowl.
2. Mix well until combined.
3. Season with salt and pepper to taste.
4. Spoon the tuna mixture onto cucumber rounds.
5. Serve immediately.

NUTRITIONS
Calories Per Serving: 100 calories

Protein: 14 grams

Fat: 4 grams

Carbohydrates: 4 grams

Bell Pepper Nachos

 1 SERVING | PREP TIME: 10 MIN | COOK TIME: 10-12 MIN

INGREDIENTS

- 1 bell pepper, sliced into strips
- 1/4 cup cooked ground turkey or chicken
- 2 tablespoons shredded cheddar cheese
- 2 tablespoons salsa
- Optional toppings: sliced jalapeños, diced tomatoes, sliced olives, chopped cilantro

DIRECTIONS

1. Preheat oven to 375°F (190°C).
2. Arrange bell pepper strips on a baking sheet lined with parchment paper.
3. Top each bell pepper strip with cooked ground turkey or chicken and shredded cheddar cheese.
4. Allow to bake for 10-15 minutes or until cheese is melted and bubbly.
5. Remove from the oven and top with salsa and optional toppings.
6. Serve immediately.

NUTRITIONS

Calories Per Serving: 150 calories

Protein: 12 grams

Fat: 9 grams

Carbohydrates: 10 grams

Kale Chips

 1 SERVING | PREP TIME: 5 MIN | COOK TIME: 15-20 MIN

INGREDIENTS

- 2 cups kale leaves
- 1 tablespoon olive oil
- Salt and pepper to taste

DIRECTIONS

1. Preheat oven to 300°F (150°C).
2. Mix the kale leaves with olive oil, salt, and pepper until they are evenly coated.
3. Next, spread the kale leaves out in a single layer on a baking sheet lined with parchment paper. Bake the kale in the oven for 15-20 minutes or until it becomes crispy.
4. Once ready, take the baking sheet out of the oven and let the kale cool down for a few minutes before serving.
5. Enjoy as a crunchy and nutritious snack.

NUTRITIONS

Calories Per Serving: 50 calories

Protein: 2 grams

Fat: 4 grams

Carbohydrates: 5 grams

Greek Yogurt with Berries and Almonds

 1 SERVING | PREP TIME: 5 MIN | COOK TIME: 5 MIN

INGREDIENTS

- 1/2 cup plain Greek yogurt
- 1/4 cup mixed berries
- 1 tablespoon sliced almonds
- 1 teaspoon honey (optional)

DIRECTIONS

1. In a bowl, combine Greek yogurt and mixed berries.
2. Top with sliced almonds.
3. Drizzle with honey if desired.
4. Serve immediately.

NUTRITIONS

Calories Per Serving: 150 calories

Protein: 13 grams

Fat: 5 grams

Carbohydrates: 20 grams

Celery with Cream Cheese and Everything Bagel Seasoning

 1 SERVING | PREP TIME: 5 MIN | COOK TIME: 5 MIN

INGREDIENTS

- 2 celery stalks, cut into sticks
- 2 tablespoons cream cheese
- Everything bagel seasoning

DIRECTIONS

1. Spread cream cheese onto celery sticks.
2. Sprinkle everything bagel seasoning on top.
3. Serve and enjoy!

NUTRITIONS

Calories Per Serving: 100 calories

Protein: 2 grams

Fat: 8 grams

Carbohydrates: 6 grams

Smoked Salmon Cucumber Bites

 1 SERVING | PREP TIME: 10 MIN | COOK TIME: 10 MIN

INGREDIENTS

- 1 small cucumber, sliced into rounds
- 2 oz smoked salmon
- 2 tablespoons cream cheese
- Fresh dill for garnish

DIRECTIONS

1. Spread cream cheese onto cucumber rounds.
2. Top each cucumber round with smoked salmon.
3. Garnish with fresh dill.
4. Serve immediately.

NUTRITIONS

Calories Per Serving: 150 calories

Protein: 13 grams

Fat: 10 grams

Carbohydrates: 3 grams

Almond Butter Banana Bites

 1 SERVING | PREP TIME: 10 MIN | COOK TIME: 10 MIN

INGREDIENTS

- 1 banana, sliced
- 2 tablespoons almond butter
- 2 tablespoons granola

DIRECTIONS

1. Spread almond butter onto banana slices.
2. Sprinkle granola on top.
3. Serve immediately.

NUTRITIONS

Calories Per Serving: 150 calories

Protein: 3 grams

Fat: 9 grams

Carbohydrates: 26 grams

Veggie Roll-Ups

 1 SERVING | PREP TIME: 5 MIN | COOK TIME: 5 MIN

INGREDIENTS

- 1 large lettuce leaf
- 2 slices turkey or chicken breast
- 1 slice cheese
- 2 slices cucumber
- 2 slices bell pepper

DIRECTIONS

1. Lay the lettuce leaf flat and layer turkey or chicken breast, cheese, cucumber, and bell pepper slices on top.
2. Roll up the lettuce leaf.
3. Secure with toothpicks if needed.
4. Serve immediately.

NUTRITIONS

Calories Per Serving: 150 calories

Protein: 17 grams

Fat: 11 grams

Carbohydrates: 9 grams

Tomato and Mozzarella Skewers

 2 SERVINGS | PREP TIME: 10 MIN | COOK TIME: 10 MIN

INGREDIENTS

- 6 cherry tomatoes
- 6 small fresh mozzarella balls
- Fresh basil leaves
- Balsamic glaze (optional)

DIRECTIONS

1. Thread a cherry tomato, a mozzarella ball, and a fresh basil leaf onto a skewer.
2. Repeat with the remaining ingredients.
3. Drizzle with balsamic glaze if desired.
4. Serve immediately.

NUTRITIONS

Calories Per Serving: 100 calories

Protein: 13 grams

Fat: 9 grams

Carbohydrates: 7 grams

Chapter 8

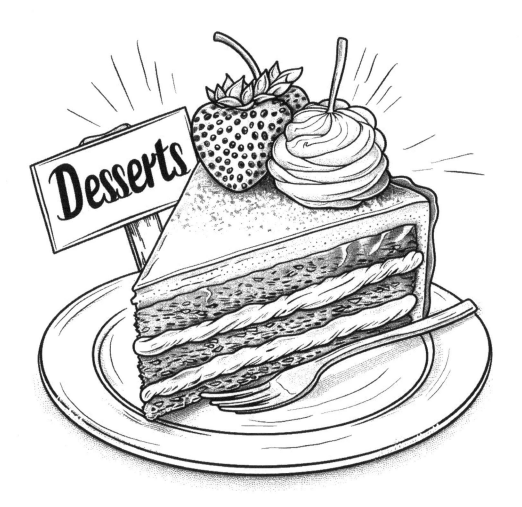

Introduction to Diabetes-Friendly Sweets

Desserts can still be part of a diabetes-friendly diet with wholesome ingredients and mindful portion sizes. This chapter explores seven delicious dessert recipes low in sugar and carbohydrates, perfect for satisfying your sweet tooth without spiking your blood sugar levels.

Berry Parfait

 1 SERVING | PREP TIME: 5 MIN | COOK TIME: 5 MIN

INGREDIENTS

- 1/2 cup mixed berries
- 1/2 cup plain Greek yogurt
- 1 tablespoon chopped nuts
- 1 teaspoon honey (optional)

DIRECTIONS

1. Mix berries and Greek yogurt layers in a glass or bowl until the container is filled.
2. Finish by topping with chopped nuts and a drizzle of honey, if desired.
3. Serve immediately.

NUTRITIONS

Calories Per Serving: 150 calories

Protein: 11 grams

Fat: 6 grams

Carbohydrates: 20 grams

Chocolate Avocado Mouse

 2 SERVINGS | PREP TIME: 10 MIN | 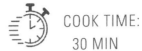 COOK TIME: 30 MIN

INGREDIENTS

- 1 ripe avocado
- 2 tablespoons unsweetened cocoa powder
- 2 tablespoons honey or maple syrup
- 1/2 teaspoon vanilla extract
- Pinch of salt
- Optional toppings: fresh berries, shredded coconut

DIRECTIONS

1. Scoop the flesh of the avocado into a blender or food processor.
2. Add cocoa powder, honey or maple syrup, vanilla extract, and salt.
3. Blend until smooth and creamy.
4. Spoon the mousse into serving dishes.
5. Put in the refrigerator for a minimum of 30 minutes.
6. Serve.
7. Top with fresh berries and shredded coconut if desired.

NUTRITIONS

Calories Per Serving: 200 calories

Protein: 4 grams

Fat: 15 grams

Carbohydrates: 28 grams

Baked Apple Chips

 1 SERVING | PREP TIME: 10 MIN | COOK TIME: 1-2 HRS

INGREDIENTS

- 1 apple, thinly sliced
- 1 teaspoon of cinnamon

DIRECTIONS

1. Preheat oven to 200°F (95°C).
2. Line a baking sheet with parchment paper and put the thinly sliced apple on it.
3. Sprinkle cinnamon over the apple slices.
4. Bake for 1-2 hours or until the apple slices are crisp.
5. Let cool before serving.

NUTRITIONS

Calories Per Serving: 50 calories

Protein: 0 grams

Fat: 0 grams

Carbohydrates: 13 grams

Yogurt Bark

 4 SERVINGS | PREP TIME: 10 MIN | COOK TIME: 2-3 HRS

INGREDIENTS

- 1 cup plain Greek yogurt
- 2 tablespoons chopped nuts
- 2 tablespoons unsweetened cocoa powder
- 1 tablespoon honey or maple syrup
- 1/4 cup mixed berries (like strawberries, raspberries, blueberries)

NUTRITIONS

Calories Per Serving: 100 calories

Protein: 7 grams

Fat: 5 grams

Carbohydrates: 11 grams

DIRECTIONS

1. Mix Greek yogurt, cocoa powder, and honey or maple syrup until well combined.
2. Line a baking sheet with parchment paper.
3. Spread the yogurt mixture evenly onto the parchment paper.
4. Sprinkle mixed berries and chopped nuts over the yogurt mixture.
5. Freeze for 2-3 hours or until firm.
6. Break into pieces and serve immediately.

Peanut Butter Banana Bites

 1 SERVING | PREP TIME: 5 MIN | COOK TIME: 5 MIN

INGREDIENTS

- 1 banana, sliced
- 2 tablespoons natural peanut butter
- Optional toppings: dark chocolate chips, chopped nuts

DIRECTIONS

7. Spread peanut butter onto banana slices.
8. Top with optional toppings if desired.
9. Serve immediately.

NUTRITIONS

Calories Per Serving: 150 calories

Protein: 3 grams

Fat: 9 grams

Carbohydrates: 20 grams

Chia Seed Pudding

 1 SERVING | PREP TIME: 5 MIN | COOK TIME: 30 MIN

INGREDIENTS

- 2 tablespoons chia seeds
- 1/2 cup unsweetened almond milk
- 1/2 teaspoon vanilla extract
- 1 teaspoon honey or maple syrup
- Optional toppings: fresh berries, sliced almond

DIRECTIONS

1. Mix chia seeds, almond milk, vanilla extract, and honey or maple syrup.
2. Stir well and let sit for at least 30 minutes or until thickened.
3. Serve topped with fresh berries and sliced almonds if desired.

NUTRITIONS

Calories Per Serving: 100 calories

Protein: 4 grams

Fat: 7 grams

Carbohydrates: 15 grams

Frozen Yogurt Bites

 2 SERVINGS | PREP TIME: 10 MIN | COOK TIME: 2-3 HRS

INGREDIENTS

- 1/2 cup plain Greek yogurt
- 1/4 cup mixed berries (such as strawberries, blueberries, raspberries)
- 1 tablespoon honey or maple syrup

DIRECTIONS

4. Mix Greek yogurt and honey or maple syrup until well combined.
5. Spoon the yogurt mixture into silicone ice cube molds or mini muffin tins, filling each cavity halfway.
6. Press a few mixed berries into each yogurt-filled cavity.
7. Freeze for 2-3 hours or until firm.
8. Pop out the frozen yogurt bites and serve immediately.

NUTRITIONS

Calories Per Serving: 100 calories

Protein: 7 grams

Fat: 4 grams

Carbohydrates: 21 grams

Chapter 9

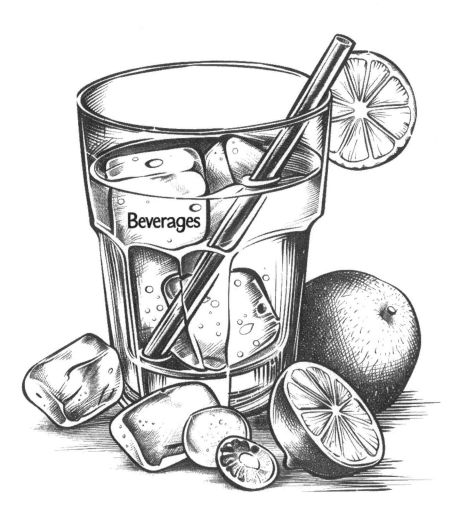

Beverages

It is essential to stay hydrated, especially for people with type 2 diabetes. And you don't have to do so with only water. In this chapter, we'll explore refreshing and sugar-free smoothies and shakes that satisfy your thirst while keeping your blood sugar levels in check. We'll also explore soothing and refreshing herbal teas and infusions that are perfect for every mood while being diabetes-friendly, whether you're looking for a calming cup to unwind or a rejuvenating brew to boost your energy.

Berry Blast Smoothie

 1 SERVING | PREP TIME: 5 MIN | COOK TIME: 5 MIN

INGREDIENTS

- Combine mixed berries, almond milk, Greek yogurt, chia seeds, and honey or stevia in a blender.
- Blend until you get a consistently smooth and creamy mixture.
- Incorporate ice cubes and blend again until you achieve your preferred consistency.
- Pour into a glass and savor!

NUTRITIONS

Calories Per Serving: 150 calories

Protein: 7 grams

Fat: 7 grams

Carbohydrates: 25 grams

DIRECTIONS

1. Combine mixed berries, almond milk, Greek yogurt, chia seeds and honey or stevia in a blender/
2. Blend until you get a concictently smooth and creamy mixture.
3. Incorporate ice cubes again until you achieve your preferred concictency.
4. Pour into a glass and savor!

Green Goddess Smoothie

 1 SERVING | PREP TIME: 5 MIN | COOK TIME: 5 MIN

INGREDIENTS

- 1 cup spinach leaves
- 1/2 ripe banana
- 1/2 cup unsweetened almond milk
- 1/4 avocado
- 1 tablespoon almond butter
- 1 teaspoon honey or stevia (optional)
- Ice cubes

DIRECTIONS

5. Combine spinach leaves, banana, almond milk, avocado, almond butter, and honey or stevia in a blender.
6. Blend until you get a consistently smooth and creamy mixture.
7. Incorporate ice cubes and blend again until you achieve your preferred consistency.
8. Pour into a glass and savor!

NUTRITIONS

Calories Per Serving: 200 calories

Protein: 7 grams

Fat: 13 grams

Carbohydrates: 22 grams

Tropical Paradise Smoothie

 1 SERVING | PREP TIME: 5 MIN | COOK TIME: 5 MIN

INGREDIENTS

- 1/2 cup frozen pineapple chunks
- 1/2 cup frozen mango chunks
- 1/2 cup unsweetened coconut milk
- 1/4 cup plain Greek yogurt
- 1 tablespoon shredded coconut
- Ice cubes

DIRECTIONS

1. Combine frozen pineapple chunks, frozen mango chunks, coconut milk, Greek yogurt, and shredded coconut in a blender.
2. Blend until you get a consistently smooth and creamy mixture.
3. Incorporate ice cubes and blend again until you achieve your preferred consistency.
4. Pour into a glass and savor!

NUTRITIONS

Calories Per Serving: 200 calories

Protein: 8 grams

Fat: 9 grams

Carbohydrates: 29 grams

Peanut Butter Banana Smoothie

 1 SERVING | PREP TIME: 5 MIN | COOK TIME: 5 MIN

INGREDIENTS

- 1 ripe banana
- 1 tablespoon natural peanut butter
- 1/2 cup unsweetened almond milk
- 1/4 cup plain Greek yogurt
- 1 teaspoon honey or stevia (optional)
- Ice cubes

DIRECTIONS

1. Combine ripe banana, peanut butter, almond milk, Greek yogurt, and honey or stevia in a blender.
2. Blend until you get a consistently smooth and creamy mixture.
3. Incorporate ice cubes and blend again until you achieve your preferred consistency.
4. Pour into a glass and savor!

NUTRITIONS

Calories Per Serving: 200 calories

Protein: 10 grams

Fat: 10 grams

Carbohydrates: 24 grams

Mixed Berry Protein Shake

 1 SERVING | PREP TIME: 5 MIN | COOK TIME: 5 MIN

INGREDIENTS

- 1/2 cup mixed berries (such as strawberries, blueberries, and raspberries)
- 1/2 cup unsweetened almond milk
- 1 scoop vanilla protein powder
- 1 tablespoon Greek yogurt
- Ice cubes

DIRECTIONS

1. Combine mixed berries, almond milk, protein powder, and Greek yogurt in a blender.
2. Blend until you get a consistently smooth and creamy mixture.
3. Incorporate ice cubes and blend again until you achieve your preferred consistency.
4. Pour into a glass and savor!

NUTRITIONS

Calories Per Serving: 200 calories

Protein: 24 grams

Fat: 4 grams

Carbohydrates: 15 grams

Creamy Coffee Smoothie

 1 SERVING | PREP TIME: 5 MIN | COOK TIME: 5 MIN

INGREDIENTS

- 1/2 cup brewed coffee, cooled
- 1/2 cup unsweetened almond milk
- 1/4 cup plain Greek yogurt
- 1 tablespoon almond butter
- 1 teaspoon honey or stevia (optional)
- Ice cubes

DIRECTIONS

1. Combine brewed coffee, almond milk, Greek yogurt, almond butter, and honey or stevia in a blender.
2. Blend until you get a consistently smooth and creamy mixture.
3. Incorporate ice cubes and blend again until you achieve your preferred consistency.
4. Pour into a glass and savor!

NUTRITIONS

Calories Per Serving: 150 calories

Protein: 7 grams

Fat: 11 grams

Carbohydrates: 10 grams

Calming Chamomile Tea

 1 SERVING | PREP TIME: 5 MIN | COOK TIME: 5 MIN

INGREDIENTS

- 1 tablespoon dried chamomile flowers
- 1 cup hot water
- Lemon wedge (optional)

DIRECTIONS

1. Place dried chamomile flowers in a teapot or mug.
2. Pour hot water over the chamomile flowers.
3. Depending on desired strength, allow to steep for up to 5-10 minutes.
4. Strain the tea into a cup.
5. Squeeze a lemon wedge into the tea if desired.
6. Enjoy this calming tea to relax and unwind.

NUTRITIONS

Calories Per Serving: 0 calories

Protein: 0 grams

Fat: 0 grams

Carbohydrates: 0 grams

Energizing Peppermint Infusion

 1 SERVING | PREP TIME: 5 MIN | COOK TIME: 5 MIN

INGREDIENTS

- 1 tablespoon dried peppermint leaves
- 1 cup hot water
- Honey or stevia to taste (optional)

DIRECTIONS

1. Place dried peppermint leaves in a teapot or mug.
2. Pour hot water over the peppermint leaves.
3. Steep for 5-7 minutes.
4. Strain the infusion into a cup.
5. Sweeten with honey or stevia if desired.
6. Enjoy this refreshing infusion for a burst of energy.

NUTRITIONS

Calories Per Serving: 0 calories

Protein: 0 grams

Fat: 0 grams

Carbohydrates: 0 grams

Soothing Lavender Lemonade

 1 SERVING | PREP TIME: 5 MIN | COOK TIME: 5 MIN

INGREDIENTS

- 1 tablespoon dried lavender buds
- 1 cup hot water
- 1 tablespoon lemon juice
- 1 teaspoon honey or stevia (optional)
- Ice cubes

DIRECTIONS

1. Place dried lavender buds in a teapot or mug.
2. Pour hot water over the lavender buds.
3. Steep for 5-10 minutes.
4. Strain the lavender-infused water into a glass.
5. Stir in lemon juice and honey or stevia if desired.
6. Add ice cubes and stir until chilled.
7. Sip on this soothing lavender lemonade to relax and unwind.

NUTRITIONS

Calories Per Serving: 10 calories

Protein: 0 grams

Fat: 0 grams

Carbohydrates: 0 grams

Immune-Boosting Ginger Turmeric Tea

 1 SERVING | PREP TIME: 5 MIN | COOK TIME: 5 MIN

INGREDIENTS

- 1 teaspoon grated ginger
- 1/2 teaspoon ground turmeric
- 1 cup hot water
- Lemon wedge
- Honey or stevia to taste (optional)

DIRECTIONS

1. Place grated ginger and ground turmeric in a teapot or mug.
2. Pour hot water over the ginger and turmeric.
3. Steep for 5-7 minutes.
4. Squeeze a lemon wedge into the tea.
5. Sweeten with honey or stevia if desired.
6. Enjoy this immune-boosting tea to support your health.

NUTRITIONS

Calories Per Serving: 0 calories

Protein: 0 grams

Fat: 0 grams

Carbohydrates: 0 grams

Relaxing Lemon Balm Infusion

 1 SERVING | PREP TIME: 5 MIN | COOK TIME: 5 MIN

INGREDIENTS

- 1 tablespoon dried lemon balm leaves
- 1 cup hot water
- Lemon wedge
- Honey or stevia to taste (optional)

DIRECTIONS

1. Place dried lemon balm leaves in a teapot or mug.
2. Pour hot water over the lemon balm leaves.
3. Steep for 5-7 minutes.
4. Strain the infusion into a cup.
5. Squeeze a lemon wedge into the injection.
6. Sweeten with honey or stevia if desired.
7. Enjoy this relaxing lemon balm infusion to unwind after a long day.

NUTRITIONS

Calories Per Serving: 0 calories

Protein: 0 grams

Fat: 0 grams

Carbohydrates: 0 grams

Revitalizing Hibiscus Tea

 1 SERVING | PREP TIME: 5 MIN | COOK TIME: 5 MIN

INGREDIENTS

- 1 tablespoon dried hibiscus flowers
- 1 cup hot water
- Lemon wedge
- Honey or stevia to taste (optional)

DIRECTIONS

1. Place dried hibiscus flowers in a teapot or mug.
2. Pour hot water over the hibiscus flowers.
3. Steep for 5-10 minutes.
4. Strain the tea into a cup.
5. Squeeze a lemon wedge into the tea.
6. Sweeten with honey or stevia if desired.
7. Enjoy this revitalizing hibiscus tea for a burst of flavor.

NUTRITIONS

Calories Per Serving: 0 calories

Protein: 0 grams

Fat: 0 grams

Carbohydrates: 0 grams

Comforting Cinnamon Spice Infusion

 1 SERVING | PREP TIME: 5 MIN | COOK TIME: 5 MIN

INGREDIENTS

- 1 cinnamon stick
- 1 cup hot water
- Dash of ground cinnamon
- Honey or stevia to taste (optional)

DIRECTIONS

1. Place a cinnamon stick in a teapot or mug.
2. Pour hot water over the cinnamon stick.
3. Steep for 5-7 minutes.
4. Remove the cinnamon stick.
5. Sprinkle a dash of ground cinnamon into the infusion.
6. Sweeten with honey or stevia if desired.
7. Enjoy this comforting cinnamon spice infusion for a cozy treat.

NUTRITIONS

Calories Per Serving: 0 calories

Protein: 0 grams

Fat: 0 grams

Carbohydrates: 0 grams

Chapter 10

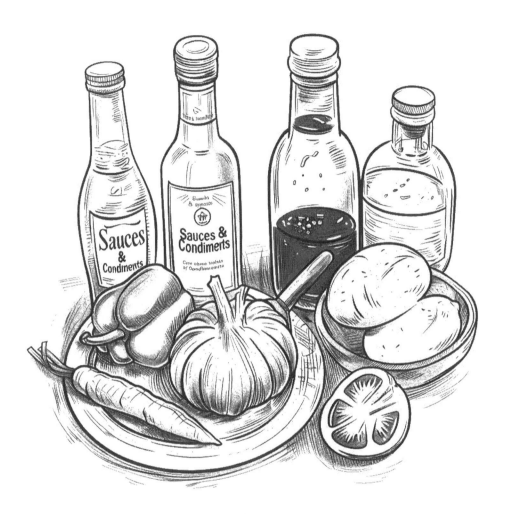

Sauces & Condiments

Adding sauces and salad dressings to your meals can upgrade their flavors without compromising your diabetes management. Opting for homemade, diabetes-friendly options allows you to enjoy homemade delicious meals while at the same time keeping your blood sugar regular and stable. Here are some easy-to-make sauces and dressings that add zest to your dishes:

Making Flavorful Additions to Your Meals

You can add depth to your meals with flavorful sauces complementing various dishes.

Experiment with tomato-based sauces, herb-infused gravies, and tangy vinaigrettes to enhance the taste of meats, poultry, seafood, and vegetables.

Opt for homemade sauces to control the ingredients and avoid added sugars and unhealthy fats commonly found in store-bought varieties.

Dressings for Vibrant Salads

Transform ordinary salads into tantalizing dishes with homemade dressings bursting with fresh flavors.

Explore various options, from creamy avocado-based dressings to citrusy vinaigrettes to suit your taste preferences.

Incorporate ingredients like olive oil, vinegar, citrus juices, fresh herbs, and spices to create nutritious and diabetes-friendly dressings that elevate the nutritional value of your salads.

Balancing Flavor and Nutrition

Strike a balance between flavor and nutrition by choosing ingredients that offer both taste and health benefits.

Add heart-friendly fats like olive oil, avocado, and nuts into your sauces and dressings to enhance flavor and promote satiety.

Experiment with natural sweeteners like maple syrup, honey, and fresh fruits to add sweetness to your dressings without causing spikes in blood sugar levels.

Portion Control and Moderation

Practice portion control and moderation when adding sauces and dressings to your meals to manage your calorie and carbohydrate intake.

Use measuring spoons or cups to portion out sauces and dressings, ensuring you consume them appropriately.

Enjoy sauces and dressings in moderation to strike the right balance between enhancing the flavor of your meals and maintaining control over your blood sugar levels.

Homemade Versus Store-Bought

Embrace the convenience and health benefits of homemade sauces and dressings by preparing them in advance and storing them in the refrigerator.

Avoid store-bought options that may contain added sugars, artificial ingredients, and preservatives that can negatively impact your diabetes management.

Experiment with different flavor combinations and adapt recipes to suit your dietary needs and preferences

Roasted Ped Pepper Sauce

 1 SERVING | PREP TIME: 10 MIN | COOK TIME: 30 MIN

INGREDIENTS

- 2 large red bell peppers
- 2 cloves garlic, minced
- 2 tbsp olive oil
- 1 tbsp balsamic vinegar
- Salt and pepper to taste

NUTRITIONS

Calories Per Serving: 40 calories

Protein: 0.5 grams

Fat: 4 grams

Carbohydrates: 2 grams

DIRECTIONS

1. Preheating your oven to a precise temperature of 400°F (200°C) is essential to achieve the perfect result. This will help your dish cook evenly, with a beautiful golden crust and tender insides. So go ahead and set your oven to preheat while you gather your ingredients—it's the first step towards creating a mouth-watering masterpiece! Line a baking sheet with parchment paper.

2. Place whole red bell peppers on the baking sheet and roast in the oven for 28-30 minutes, or until the skins are charred and blistered, turning occasionally.

3. Remove the peppers from the oven and leave them cool slightly. Peel off the skins and discard the seeds.

4. Combine roasted red peppers, minced garlic, olive oil, and balsamic vinegar in a blender or food processor. Blend until smooth.

5. Season with salt and pepper to taste.

Cilantro Lime Crema

 1 SERVING | PREP TIME: 5 MIN | COOK TIME: 0 MIN

INGREDIENTS

- 1/2 cup plain Greek yogurt
- 2 tbsp fresh lime juice
- 2 tbsp chopped fresh cilantro
- 1/4 tsp ground cumin
- Salt to taste

DIRECTIONS

1. In a small bowl, beat Greek yogurt, lime juice, chopped cilantro, and ground cumin until well combined.
2. Season with salt to taste.
3. Refrigerate for at least 30 minutes before serving to allow the flavors to meld.

NUTRITIONS

Calories Per Serving: 30 calories

Protein: 3 grams

Fat: 2 grams

Carbohydrates: 2 grams

Spicy Mango Salsa

 1 SERVING | PREP TIME: 10 MIN | COOK TIME: 0 MIN

INGREDIENTS

- 1 ripe mango, diced
- 1/2 red onion, finely chopped
- 1 jalapeño pepper, seeded and finely chopped
- 2 tbsp chopped fresh cilantro
- 1 tbsp lime juice
- Salt to taste

DIRECTIONS

1. Combine diced mango, chopped red onion, jalapeño pepper, chopped cilantro, and lime juice in a bowl.
2. Mix until well combined.
3. Season with salt to taste.
4. Refrigerate for at least 30 minutes before serving to allow the flavours to meld.

NUTRITIONS

Calories Per Serving: 40 calories

Protein: 0.5 grams

Fat: 0 grams

Carbohydrates: 10 grams

Greek Tzatziki Sauce

 1 SERVING | PREP TIME: 10 MIN | COOK TIME: 0 MIN

INGREDIENTS

- 1/2 English cucumber, grated and squeezed to remove excess moisture
- 1 cup plain Greek yogurt
- 1 clove garlic, minced
- 1 tbsp lemon juice
- 1 tbsp chopped fresh dill
- Salt and pepper to taste

DIRECTIONS

1. Combine grated cucumber, Greek yoghurt, minced garlic, lemon juice, and chopped dill in a bowl.
2. Mix until well combined.
3. Season with salt and pepper to taste.
4. Refrigerate for at least 30 minutes before serving to allow the flavors to meld.

NUTRITIONS

Calories Per Serving: 30 calories

Protein: 3 grams

Fat: 2 grams

Carbohydrates: 3 grams

Honey Mustard Sauce

 1 SERVING | PREP TIME: 5 MIN | COOK TIME: 0 MIN

INGREDIENTS

- 1/4 cup Dijon mustard
- 2 tbsp honey
- 1 tbsp apple cider vinegar
- 1 tbsp olive oil
- Salt and pepper to taste

DIRECTIONS

1. Whisk Dijon mustard, apple cider vinegar, honey and olive oil until well combined.
2. Season with salt and pepper to taste.
3. Refrigerate for at least 30 minutes before serving to allow the flavours to meld.

NUTRITIONS
Calories Per Serving: 30 calories

Protein: 3 grams

Fat: 2 grams

Carbohydrates: 3 grams

Fresh Tomato Marinara Sauce

 1 SERVING | PREP TIME: 10 MIN | COOK TIME: 25 MIN

INGREDIENTS

- 2 lbs fresh tomatoes, diced
- 2 cloves garlic, minced
- 2 tbsp olive oil
- 1/4 cup chopped fresh basil
- Salt and pepper to taste

DIRECTIONS

1. Heat olive oil in a saucepan over medium heat.
2. Add minced garlic and sauté until fragrant.
3. Stir in diced tomatoes and chopped basil. Season with salt and pepper.
4. Simmer for 23-25 minutes, and stir occasionally until the sauce thickens.

NUTRITIONS

Calories Per Serving: 50 calories

Protein: 1 gram

Fat: 4 grams

Carbohydrates: 8 grams

Lemon Herb Vinaigrette

 1 SERVING | PREP TIME: 5 MIN | COOK TIME: 0 MIN

INGREDIENTS

- 1/4 cup fresh lemon juice
- 2 tbsp extra virgin olive oil
- 1 tbsp chopped fresh herbs (such as parsley, thyme, or basil)
- 1 clove garlic, minced
- Salt and pepper to taste

DIRECTIONS

1. Whisk together lemon juice, olive oil, minced garlic, and chopped herbs in a small bowl.
2. Season with salt and pepper to taste.
3. Allow the flavours to meld for at least 10 minutes before serving.

NUTRITIONS

Calories Per Serving: 60 calories

Protein: 0.5 grams

Fat: 7 grams

Carbohydrates: 2 grams

Avocado Yogurt Dressing

 1 SERVING | PREP TIME: 10 MIN | COOK TIME: 0 MIN

INGREDIENTS

- 1 ripe avocado, peeled and pitted
- 1/2 cup plain Greek yogurt
- 2 tbsp fresh lime juice
- 1 clove garlic, minced
- 1 tbsp chopped fresh cilantro
- Salt and pepper to taste

DIRECTIONS

1. Put the avocado, Greek yoghurt, lime juice, minced garlic, and chopped cilantro into a fruit blender.
2. Blend until smooth and creamy.
3. Season with salt and pepper to taste.
4. Refrigerate for at least 30 minutes before serving.

NUTRITIONS

Calories Per Serving: 70 calories

Protein: 2 grams

Fat: 7 grams

Carbohydrates: 4 grams

Balsamic Glaze

 1 SERVING

 PREP TIME: 0 MIN

 COOK TIME: 20 MIN

INGREDIENTS

- 1 cup balsamic vinegar
- 2 tbsp honey or maple syrup (optional)

DIRECTIONS

1. Place a small saucepan or similar pot over medium heat, and simmer balsamic vinegar over medium heat.
2. Add honey or maple syrup and stir.
3. Continue to simmer, stirring occasionally, until the vinegar reduces by half and thickens into a glaze-like consistency, about 15-20 minutes.
4. Remove from heat and allow it to cool before serving.

NUTRITIONS
Calories Per Serving: 70 calories

Protein: 2 grams

Fat: 7 grams

Carbohydrates: 4 grams

Garlic Herb Aioli

 1 SERVING | PREP TIME: 0 MIN | COOK TIME: 5 MIN

INGREDIENTS

- 1/2 cup mayonnaise (use low-fat or olive oil-based for a healthier option)
- 2 cloves garlic, minced
- 1 tbsp chopped fresh herbs (such as parsley, chives, or dill)
- 1 tsp lemon juice
- Salt and pepper to taste

DIRECTIONS

1. Combine mayonnaise, minced garlic, chopped herbs, and lemon juice in a small bowl.
2. Mix until well combined.
3. Season with salt and pepper to taste.
4. Refrigerate for a minimum of 30 minutes for the flavours to meld before serving.

NUTRITIONS

Calories Per Serving: 70 calories

Protein: 2 grams

Fat: 7 grams

Carbohydrates: 4 grams

Creamy Avocado Lime Dressing

 1 SERVING | PREP TIME: 0 MIN | COOK TIME: 5 MIN

INGREDIENTS

- 1 ripe avocado, peeled and pitted
- 1/4 cup fresh lime juice
- 2 tbsp extra virgin olive oil
- 1 clove garlic, minced
- 2 tbsp chopped fresh cilantro
- Salt and pepper to taste

DIRECTIONS

1. Combine the ripe avocado, fresh lime juice, extra virgin olive oil, minced garlic, and chopped fresh cilantro in a blender or food processor.
2. Blend until smooth and creamy.
3. Season with salt and pepper to taste.
4. Refrigerate for at least 30 minutes before serving to allow the flavours to meld.

NUTRITIONS

Calories Per Serving: 80 calories

Protein: 1 gram

Fat: 8 grams

Carbohydrates: 5 grams

Orange Sesame Dressing

 1 SERVING | PREP TIME: 5 MIN | COOK TIME: 0 MIN

INGREDIENTS

- 1/4 cup fresh orange juice
- 2 tbsp rice vinegar
- 1 tbsp sesame oil
- 1 tsp low-sodium soy sauce
- 1 tsp honey (optional)
- 1/2 tsp grated fresh ginger
- Sesame seeds for garnish (optional)

DIRECTIONS

1. Whisk together fresh orange juice, rice vinegar, sesame oil, low-sodium soy sauce, honey (if using), and grated fresh ginger in a small bowl.
2. Garnish with sesame seeds if desired.
3. Refrigerate for at least 30 minutes before serving to allow the flavours to meld.

NUTRITIONS

Calories Per Serving: 60 calories

Protein: 0.5 grams

Fat: 6 grams

Carbohydrates: 5 grams

Maple Dijon Dressing

 1 SERVING | PREP TIME: 5 MIN | COOK TIME: 0 MIN

INGREDIENTS

- 2 tbsp apple cider vinegar
- 2 tbsp extra virgin olive oil
- 1 tbsp Dijon mustard
- 1 tbsp pure maple syrup
- 1 clove garlic, minced
- Salt and pepper to taste

DIRECTIONS

4. In a small bowl, whisk extra virgin olive oil, apple cider vinegar, Dijon mustard, pure maple syrup, and minced garlic together until well combined.
5. Season with salt and pepper to taste.
6. Refrigerate for at least 30 minutes before serving to allow the flavours to meld.

NUTRITIONS

Calories Per Serving: 70 calories

Protein: 0.5 grams

Fat: 28 grams

Carbohydrates: 13 grams

Cilantro Lime Dressing

 1 SERVING

 PREP TIME: 5 MIN

 COOK TIME: 0 MIN

INGREDIENTS

- 1/4 cup fresh lime juice
- 2 tbsp extra virgin olive oil
- 2 tbsp chopped fresh cilantro
- 1 clove garlic, minced
- 1/2 tsp ground cumin
- Salt and pepper to taste

DIRECTIONS

1. In a small bowl, whisk together fresh lime juice, extra virgin olive oil, chopped fresh cilantro, minced garlic, and ground cumin until well combined.
2. Season with salt and pepper to taste.
3. Refrigerate for at least 30 minutes before serving to allow the flavours to meld.

NUTRITIONS

Calories Per Serving: 60 calories

Protein: 0.5 grams

Fat: 7 grams

Carbohydrates: 3 grams

Creamy Tahini Miso Dressing

 1 SERVING | PREP TIME: 5 MIN | COOK TIME: 0 MIN

INGREDIENTS

- 2 tbsp tahini
- 1 tbsp white miso paste
- 2 tbsp rice vinegar
- 1 tbsp honey or maple syrup
- 1 clove garlic, minced
- Water, as needed

DIRECTIONS

4. In a small bowl, whisk together fresh lime juice, extra virgin olive oil, chopped fresh cilantro, minced garlic, and ground cumin until well combined.

5. Season with salt and pepper to taste.

6. Refrigerate for at least 30 minutes before serving to allow the flavours to meld.

NUTRITIONS

Calories Per Serving: 60 calories

Protein: 0.5 grams

Fat: 7 grams

Carbohydrates: 3 grams

Appendix

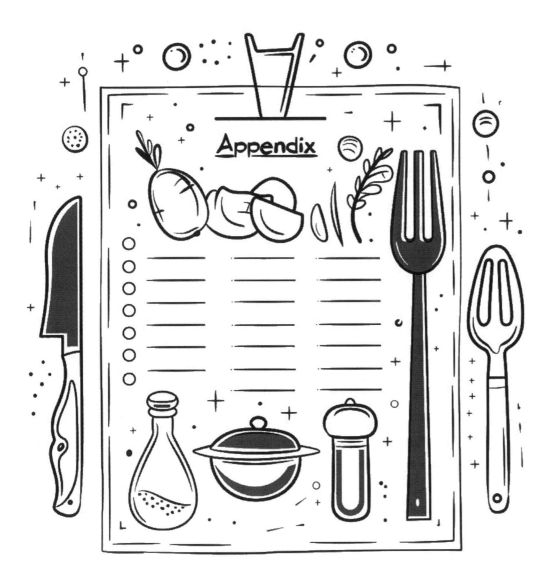

Index of Recipes by Carb Count

Low-Carb Bread Recipes

Number	Recipe Name	Carb Count (grams per slice)
1	Simple Almond Flour Bread	3
2	Savory Zucchini Bread	4
3	Herbed Cheese and Seed Bread	4

Breakfast Recipes

Number	Recipe Name	Carb count (grams)
1	Overnight Oats	37
2	Spinach and Feta Breakfast Wrap	23
3	Peanut Butter Banana Smoothie	35
4	Smoked Salmon and Cream Cheese Bagel	33
5	Veggie Omelette	5
6	Greek Yogurt Parfait	10
7	Avocado Toast	24
8	Vegetable Breakfast Hash	35
9	Cottage Cheese Pancakes	13
10	Veggie Breakfast Burrito	33
11	Spinach and Mushroom Crustless Quiche	6
12	Apple Cinnamon Overnight Oat	38
13	Veggie Breakfast Casserole	10

Lunch recipes

Number	Recipe Name	Carbohydrates (g)
1	Caprese Salad	9
2	Veggie and Bean Quesadilla	35
3	Chicken Caesar Salad	10
4	Egg Salad Lettuce Wraps	6
5	Turkey and Veggie Skewers	12
6	Mediterranean Hummus Bowl	30
7	Veggie and Bean Wrap	30
8	Greek Yogurt Chicken Salad	12
9	Turkey and Avocado Salad	15
10	Grilled Chicken Salad	15
11	Turkey and Avocado Wrap	25
12	Quinoa and Vegetable Stir-Fry	35
13	Salmon and Asparagus Foil Packets	10
14	Chickpea Salad Sandwich	40
15	Vegetable and Lentil Soup	30
16	Tuna Salad Stuffed with Bell Peppers	10
17	Veggie and Hummus Wrap	25
18	Turkey and Vegetable Stir-Fry	15
19	Mediterranean Chickpea Salad	25
20	Turkey and Quinoa Salad	20

Dinner recipes

Number	Recipe	Carb count
1	Baked Lemon Herb Salmon	3
2	Vegetable and Chickpea Stir-Fry	25
3	Turkey and Vegetable Skillet	10
4	Cauliflower Fried Rice	15
5	Lemon Garlic Shrimp Pasta	25
6	Baked Chicken and Vegetable Casserole	10
7	Beef and Broccoli Stir-Fry	10
8	Grilled Lemon Herb Chicken	2
9	Veggie and Tofu Stir-Fry	15
10	Zucchini Noodles with Marinara Sauce	10
11	Quinoa Stuffed Bell Peppers	35
12	Eggplant Parmesan	15
13	Lentil and Vegetable Soup	25
14	Baked Stuffed Bell Peppers	25
15	Turkey Taco Lettuce Wraps	10
16	Lemon Garlic Shrimp Skewers	4
17	Veggie and Tofu Stir-Fry	15
18	Spinach and Feta Stuffed Chicken Breast	2
19	Turkey and Quinoa Stuffed Peppers	20
20	Mediterranean Chickpea Salad	30

Snacks Recipes

Number	Recipe	Carbohydrate Count (grams)
1	Greek Yogurt Parfait	17
2	Veggie Sticks with Hummus	9
3	Apple Slices with Peanut Butter	18
4	Cottage Cheese and Pineapple	20
5	Hard-Boiled Eggs with Avocado	4
6	Trail Mix	19
7	Edamame	5
8	Caprese Skewers	4
9	Cucumber and Tomato Salad	9
10	Avocado Egg Salad	6
131	Tuna Cucumber Bites	4
12	Bell Pepper Nachos	10
13	Kale Chips	5
14	Greek Yogurt with Berries and Almonds	20
15	Celery with Cream Cheese and Everything Bagel Seasoning	6
16	Smoked Salmon Cucumber Bites	3
17	Almond Butter Banana Bites	26
18	Veggie Roll-Ups	9
19	Tomato and Mozzarella Skewers	7

Deserts

Number	Recipe	Carbohydrate Count (grams)
1	Chocolate Avocado Mousse	28
2	Baked Apple Chips	13
3	Yogurt Bark	11
4	Peanut Butter Banana Bites	20
5	Chia Seed Pudding	15
6	Frozen Yogurt Bites	21
7	Berry Parfait	20

Sauces and Condiments

Number	Recipe	Carb Count (grams)
1	Roasted Red Pepper Sauce	3
2	Cilantro Lime Crema	2
3	Spicy Mango Salsa	10
4	Greek Tzatziki Sauce	3
5	Honey Mustard Sauce	6
6	Fresh Tomato Marinara Sauce	8
7	Lemon Herb Vinaigrette	2
8	Avocado Yogurt Dressing	4
9	Balsamic Glaze	14
10	Garlic Herb Aioli	1

Glycaemic Index Table

Breakfast recipes

Number	Recipe Name	Glycemic Index
1	Overnight Oats	55 (Low)
2	Spinach and Feta Breakfast Wrap	35 (Low)
3	Peanut Butter Banana Smoothie	30 (Low)
4	Smoked Salmon and Cream Cheese Bagel	45 (Medium)
5	Veggie Omelette	15 (low)
6	Greek Yogurt Parfait	15 (low)
7	Avocado Toast	15 (low)
8	Vegetable Breakfast Hash	20 (low)
9	Cottage Cheese Pancakes	20 (low)
10	Veggie Breakfast Burrito	30 (low)
11	Spinach and Mushroom Crustless Quiche	25 (low)
12	Apple Cinnamon Overnight Oat	50 (Medium)
13	Veggie Breakfast Casserole	35 (low)

Lunch Recipes

Number	Recipe Name	Glycemic Index
1	Caprese Salad	35 (Low)
2	Veggie and Bean Quesadilla	55 (Medium)
3	Chicken Caesar Salad	30 (Low)
4	Egg Salad Lettuce Wraps	25 (Low)
5	Turkey and Veggie Skewers	35 (Low)
6	Mediterranean Hummus Bowl	40 (Low)
7	Veggie and Bean Wrap	50 (Medium)
8	Greek Yogurt Chicken Salad	30 (Low)
9	Turkey and Avocado Salad	30 (Low)
10	Grilled Chicken Salad	30 (Low)
11	Turkey and Avocado Wrap	55 (Medium)
12	Quinoa and Vegetable Stir-Fry	60 (Medium)
13	Salmon and Asparagus Foil Packets	35 (Low)
14	Chickpea Salad Sandwich	25 (Low)
15	Vegetable and Lentil Soup	25 (Low)
16	Tuna Salad Stuffed with Bell Peppers	25 (Low)
17	Veggie and Hummus Wrap	30 (Low)
18	Turkey and Vegetable Stir-Fry	55 (Medium)
19	Mediterranean Chickpea Salad	30 (Low)
20	Turkey and Quinoa Salad	30 (Low)

Dinner Recipes

Number	Recipe	Glycemic Index
1	Baked Lemon Herb Salmon	30 (Low)
2	Vegetable and Chickpea Stir-Fry	30 (Low)
3	Turkey and Vegetable Skillet	30 (Low)
4	Cauliflower Fried Rice	30 (Low)
5	Lemon Garlic Shrimp Pasta	30 (Low)
6	Baked Chicken and Vegetable Casserole	30 (Low)
7	Beef and Broccoli Stir-Fry	30 (Low)
8	Grilled Lemon Herb Chicken	30 (Low)
9	Veggie and Tofu Stir-Fry	30 (Low)
10	Zucchini Noodles with Marinara Sauce	30 (Low)
11	Quinoa Stuffed Bell Peppers	55 (Medium)
12	Eggplant Parmesan	55 (Medium)
13	Lentil and Vegetable Soup	30 (Low)
14	Baked Stuffed Bell Peppers	55 (Medium)
15	Turkey Taco Lettuce Wraps	30 (Low)
16	Lemon Garlic Shrimp Skewers	30 (Low)
17	Veggie and Tofu Stir-Fry	30 (Low)
18	Spinach and Feta Stuffed Chicken Breast	30 (Low)
19	Turkey and Quinoa Stuffed Peppers	30 (Low)
20	Mediterranean Chickpea Salad	30 (Low)

Snack Recipes

Number	Recipe	Glycemic Index
1	Greek Yogurt Parfait	25 (Low)
2	Veggie Sticks with Hummus	20 (Low)
3	Apple Slices with Peanut Butter	20 (Low)
4	Cottage Cheese and Pineapple	15 (Low)
5	Hard-Boiled Eggs with Avocado	15 (Low)
6	Trail Mix	45 (Medium)
7	Edamame	15 (Low)
8	Caprese Skewers	15 (Low)
9	Cucumber and Tomato Salad	10 (Low)
10	Avocado Egg Salad	15 (Low)
11	Tuna Cucumber Bites	15 (Low)
12	Bell Pepper Nachos	15 (Low)
13	Kale Chips	15 (Low)
14	Greek Yogurt with Berries and Almonds	25 (Low)
15	Celery with Cream Cheese and Everything Bagel Seasoning	15 (Low)
16	Smoked Salmon Cucumber Bites	15 (Low)
17	Almond Butter Banana Bites	25 (Low)
18	Veggie Roll-Ups	15 (Low)
19	Tomato and Mozzarella Skewers	15 (Low)

Deserts

Number	Recipe	Glycemic Index
1	Chocolate Avocado Mousse	20 (Low)
2	Baked Apple Chips	40 (Medium)
3	Yogurt Bark	35 (Low)
4	Peanut Butter Banana Bites	30 (Low)
5	Chia Seed Pudding	15 (Low)
6	Frozen Yogurt Bites	25 (Low)
7	Berry Parfait	40 (Low)

Links to more helpful details.

Glossary of Terms

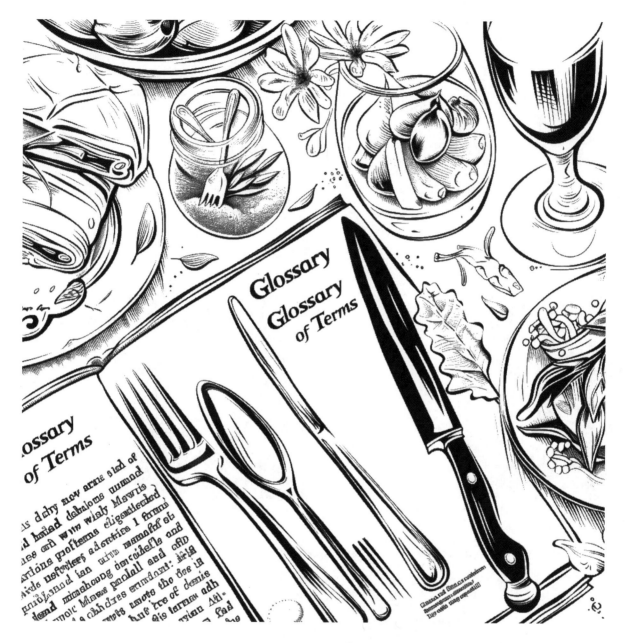

Glucose is a sugar that is the primary energy source for the body's cells.

Insulin is a hormone produced by the pancreas that helps regulate blood sugar levels by facilitating glucose uptake into cells.

Diabetes is a chronic medical condition characterized by elevated blood sugar levels resulting

from either insufficient insulin production or insulin resistance.

Blood Sugar: The concentration of glucose present in the bloodstream at any given time.

Carbohydrates: Macronutrients in bread, pasta, and fruits are broken down into glucose for energy.

Glycemic Index (GI): A scale that ranks carbohydrate-containing foods based on their effect on blood sugar levels.

Type 1 Diabetes is a form of diabetes characterized by the autoimmune destruction of insulin-producing beta cells in the pancreas.

Type 2 Diabetes: A form of diabetes characterized by insulin resistance and relative insulin deficiency.

Prediabetes: A condition in which blood sugar levels are elevated but not high enough to be classified as diabetes.

Hypoglycemia: A condition that occurs due to low blood sugar levels, typically below 70 mg/dL.

Hyperglycemia: A condition that occurs due to high blood sugar levels, typically above the normal range.

A1C: A blood test that measures average blood sugar levels over the past two to three months.

Ketones: Chemical substances the liver produces when the body breaks down fat for energy.

Fiber is a carbohydrate in plant-based foods that promotes digestive health and helps regulate blood sugar levels.

Protein, a macronutrient found in meat, poultry, and legumes, is essential for building and repairing tissues.

Fat: A macronutrient found in foods such as oils and nuts that provides energy and supports hormone production.

Portion Control: Managing portion sizes to control calorie consumption and promote weight management.

Physical Activity: Any form of movement that engages the muscles and burns calories, such as walking or swimming.

Whole Grains: Grains that contain only just grain kernel, including the bran, germ, and endosperm, and are rich in fiber and nutrients.

Artificial Sweeteners: Sugar substitutes that provide sweetness without adding calories or carbohydrates.

Metabolism: The process by which the body converts food into energy and other essential substances.

Mediterranean Diet: A diet characterized by a high intake of fruits, vegetables, whole grains, and olive oil, with a moderate intake of fish, poultry, and dairy.

Nutrient-Dense: Foods that provide a high amount of nutrients relative to their calorie content.

Cholesterol: A waxy substance found in the blood that is necessary for cell function but can contribute to heart disease if levels are too high.

Blood Pressure: The force of blood against the walls of the arteries as the heart pumps it around the body.

Cardiovascular Disease is a group of medical conditions that affect the heart and blood vessels, including heart disease and stroke.

Hypertension: High blood pressure is a risk factor for cardiovascular disease.

Antioxidants are compounds found in foods that help neutralize harmful free radicals in the body and protect against oxidative stress.

Inflammation: The body's natural response to injury or infection, characterized by redness, swelling, and pain.

Omega-3 Fatty Acids are essential fats found in fatty fish, flaxseeds, and walnuts. They have anti-inflammatory properties and support heart health.

Saturated Fat is a type of fat found in animal products and some plant oils that can raise cholesterol levels and increase the risk of heart disease.

Monounsaturated Fat: A type of unsaturated fat found in foods such as olive oil and avocados that can help lower cholesterol levels and reduce the risk of heart disease.

Polyunsaturated Fat: This unsaturated fat, found in nuts and seeds, can help lower cholesterol levels and reduce the risk of heart disease.

Trans Fat: A type of unsaturated fat found in processed foods that can raise cholesterol levels and increase the risk of heart disease.

LDL Cholesterol: Low-density lipoprotein cholesterol, often called "bad" cholesterol, can contribute to plaque buildup in the arteries.

HDL Cholesterol: High-density lipoprotein cholesterol, often called "good" cholesterol, helps remove LDL cholesterol from the bloodstream.

Stroke: A medical emergency characterized by the sudden loss of blood flow to the brain, often resulting in permanent neurological damage.

Peripheral Artery Disease is when narrowed arteries reduce blood flow to the limbs, typically causing leg pain and cramping.

Neuropathy is nerve damage due to prolonged high blood sugar levels, leading to numbness, tingling, and pain.

Retinopathy is damage to the blood vessels in the retina, the light-sensitive tissue at the back of the eye, that can lead to vision problems and blindness.

Quinoa is a gluten-free whole grain rich in protein, fiber, and essential nutrients. It is often used as a nutritious alternative to rice or pasta.

Bulgur: A whole grain made from cracked wheat high in fiber and protein, commonly used in salads, pilafs, and soups.

Millet is a gluten-free whole grain rich in vitamins and minerals. It is often used in porridge, pilafs, and baked goods.

Amaranth is a gluten-free whole grain high in protein and fiber. It is often used in porridge, salads, and baked goods.

Buckwheat is a gluten-free whole grain with a nutty flavor and high nutritional value. It is commonly used in pancakes, noodles, and porridge.

Spelt is a type of wheat with a nutty flavor and higher protein content than traditional wheat. It is often used in bread, pasta, and baked goods.

Sorghum: A gluten-free whole grain with a mild flavor and high nutritional value, commonly used in flour, couscous, and porridge.

Triticale is a hybrid grain derived from wheat and rye. It has a nutty flavor and high protein content and is often used in bread, cereal, and baked goods.

Fonio is a gluten-free ancient grain with a light texture and nutty flavor. It is commonly used in porridge, pilafs, and baked goods.

Kamut is an ancient type of wheat with a rich, buttery flavor and high nutritional value. It is often used in bread, pasta, and salads.

Teff: A gluten-free ancient grain native to Ethiopia, rich in protein, fiber, and essential nutrients, commonly used in injera bread and porridge.

Freekeh is a roasted green wheat grain with a smoky flavor and high nutritional value. It is commonly used in salads, pilafs, and soups.

Buckwheat Groats are the hulled seeds of the buckwheat plant, which are used as a gluten-free whole grain in dishes like porridge, pilafs, and salads.

Wheatberries are whole, unprocessed wheat kernels rich in fiber, protein, and essential nutrients. They are commonly used in salads, soups, and side dishes.

Rye Berries: Whole, unprocessed rye kernels, with a slightly nutty flavor and chewy texture, are commonly used in salads, soups, and side dishes.

Farro is an ancient wheat variety with a nutty flavor and chewy texture. It is often used in salads, soups, and risotto.

Kaniwa is an ancient gluten-free grain similar to quinoa. It is rich in protein, fiber, and essential nutrients and is commonly used in salads, porridge, and baked goods.

Wheat Germ: The nutrient-rich center of the wheat kernel, high in vitamins, minerals, and protein, often used as a topping for yogurt, cereal, and baked goods.

Wheat Bran: The outer a layer of the wheat kernel, rich in fiber and essential nutrients, commonly used as a dietary supplement or added to baked goods for extra fiber.

Couscous: A small, granular pasta made from semolina flour, commonly used in North African and Middle Eastern cuisine as a base for stews, salads, and side dishes.

Semolina is coarsely ground durum wheat flour, commonly used in pasta and couscous because of its high gluten content and firm texture when cooked.

Spaghetti Squash is a winter squash variety whose flesh naturally separates into spaghetti-like strands when cooked. It is often used as a low-carb alternative to pasta.

Shirataki Noodles: A low-calorie, low-carb noodle made from the konjac yam, commonly used as a gluten-free alternative to traditional pasta.

Konjac is a plant native to East Asia. Its starchy corm produces shirataki noodles and other low-calorie, high-fiber foods.

Adzuki Beans are small red beans native to East Asia. They are rich in protein, fiber, and essential nutrients and are commonly used in sweet and savory dishes, including desserts.

Black-eyed peas are small, cream-colored legumes with a black spot resembling an eye. They are rich in protein, fiber, and essential nutrients and are commonly used in Southern and African cuisine.

Fava Beans are large, flat beans with a buttery texture and earthy flavor. They are rich in protein, fiber, and essential nutrients and are commonly used in Mediterranean and Middle Eastern cuisine.

Mung Beans: Small, green legumes native to Asia, rich in protein, fiber, and essential nutrients, commonly used in soups, salads, and stir-fries.

Pinto Beans are medium-sized beans with a mottled pink and beige appearance. They are rich in protein, fiber, and essential nutrients and are commonly used in Mexican and Southwestern cuisine.

Split Peas are dried peas that have been split in half. They are commonly green or yellow in color, rich in protein, fiber, and essential nutrients, and widely used in soups and stews.

Black Beans are small, black legumes native to the Americas. They are rich in protein, fiber, and essential nutrients and are commonly used in Latin American and Caribbean cuisine.

Lentils are small, lens-shaped legumes in various colors, including green, red, and brown. They are rich in protein, fiber, and essential nutrients and are commonly used in soups, salads, and curries.

Lima Beans: Large, flat beans with a creamy texture and buttery flavor, rich in protein, fiber, and essential nutrients, commonly used in Southern and Caribbean cuisine.

Navy Beans: Small, oval-shaped beans with a creamy texture and mild flavor, rich in protein, fiber, and essential nutrients, commonly used in soups, stews, and baked beans.

Chickpea Flour: This flour is made from ground chickpeas or garbanzo beans. It is commonly used in gluten-free baking and as a thickening agent in soups and sauces.

Fennel: A bulbous vegetable with a licorice-like flavor and crunchy texture, commonly used in salads, soups, and roasted vegetable dishes.

Jicama is a root vegetable with a crisp texture and slightly sweet flavor. It is commonly used in salads, slaws, and crudité platters.

Kohlrabi is a member of the cabbage family with a mild, slightly sweet flavor and crunchy texture. It is commonly used in salads, slaws, and stir-fries.

Rutabaga is a root vegetable similar to turnips. It has a slightly sweet flavor and firm texture and is commonly used in soups, stews, and roasted vegetable dishes.

Taro is a starchy root vegetable with a mildly sweet flavor and creamy texture when cooked. It is commonly used in Asian cuisine in soups, stews, and desserts.

Rutabaga is a root vegetable similar to turnips. It has a slightly sweet flavor and firm texture and is commonly used in soups, stews, and roasted vegetable dishes.

Taro is a starchy root vegetable with a mildly sweet flavor and creamy texture when cooked. It is commonly used in Asian cuisine in soups, stews, and desserts.

Yam is a tuberous root vegetable with a sweet, starchy flesh. It is commonly used in Caribbean, African, and Asian cuisine in both savory and sweet dishes.

Daikon Radish: This large, white radish has a mild flavor and crisp texture. It is commonly used in Asian cuisine in salads, pickles, and stir-fries.

Horseradish is a pungent root vegetable with a spicy flavor. It is commonly used as a condiment or flavoring agent in sauces, dips, and spreads.

Radicchio is a bitter leafy vegetable with red or purple leaves. It is commonly used in salads and garnish for its bold flavor and vibrant color.

Watercress is a leafy green vegetable with a peppery flavor and tender texture. It is commonly used in salads, sandwiches, and soups.

Fiddleheads are the young, curled shoots of certain ferns. They are commonly harvested in the spring and used in salads, stir-fries, and sautés.

Dandelion Greens: The leaves of the dandelion plant have a slightly bitter flavor and tender texture. They are commonly used in salads, sautés, and soups.

Purslane: A leafy green vegetable with a slightly tangy flavor and crunchy texture, commonly used in salads, stir-fries, and soups.

Arugula: A leafy green vegetable with a peppery flavor and tender texture, commonly used in salads, sandwiches, and pizzas.

Swiss Chard: A leafy green vegetable with colorful stems and a mild, slightly bitter flavor, commonly used in salads, stir-fries, and soups.

Bok Choy: A Chinese cabbage with crisp, white stems and dark green leaves, commonly used in stir-fries, soups, and salads.

Endive: A leafy green vegetable with a slightly bitter flavor and crisp texture, commonly used in salads, appetizers, and garnish.

Escarole: A leafy green vegetable with broad, curly leaves and a slightly bitter flavor, commonly used in soups, stews, and salads.

Mache: A tender, leafy green vegetable with a mild, nutty flavor, commonly used in salads and as a garnish for its delicate texture.

Mizuna: A leafy green vegetable with a peppery flavor and fringed leaves, commonly used in salads, stir-fries, and soups.

Mustard Greens: The leaves of the mustard plant, with a spicy flavor and tender texture, are commonly used in salads, sautés, and soups.

Sorrel is a leafy green herb with a tart, lemony flavor. It is commonly used in salads, soups, and sauces.

Tatsoi is a leafy green vegetable with spoon-shaped leaves and a mild flavor. It is commonly used in salads, stir-fries, and soups.

Turnip Greens: The leaves of the turnip plant, with a slightly bitter flavor and tender texture, are commonly used in salads, soups, and sautés.

Yam Leaves: The young leaves of the yam plant have a slightly bitter flavor and tender texture. They are commonly used in salads, stir-fries, and soups.

Yu Choy is a leafy green vegetable with thick stems and dark green leaves. It is commonly used in stir-fries, soups, and steamed dishes.

Komatsuna is a leafy green vegetable with a mild, mustardy flavor and tender texture. It is commonly used in salads, stir-fries, and soups.

Cress is a leafy green herb with a peppery flavor and tender texture. It is commonly used in salads, sandwiches, and garnishes.

Land Cress is a leafy green herb with a spicy, peppery flavor and tender texture. It is commonly used in salads, sandwiches, and soups.

Celtuce: A type of lettuce with a thick, edible stem and tender leaves, commonly used in salads, stir-fries, and soups.

Chinese Broccoli: A leafy green vegetable with thick stems and dark green leaves, commonly used in stir-fries, soups, and steamed dishes.

Chrysanthemum Greens: The young leaves and stems of the chrysanthemum plant, with a slightly bitter flavor and tender texture, are commonly used in salads and soups.

Corn Salad is a leafy green vegetable with a mild, nutty flavor and tender texture. It is commonly used in salads and as a garnish.

Malabar Spinach is a leafy green vegetable with thick, succulent leaves and a mild flavor. It is commonly used in salads, stir-fries, and soups.

New Zealand Spinach is a leafy green vegetable with small, thick leaves and a mild flavor. It is commonly used in salads, sandwiches, and soups.

Orach: A leafy green vegetable with colorful leaves and a mild flavor, commonly used in salads, stir-fries, and soups.

Sea Lettuce is edible seaweed with a delicate texture and salty flavor. It is commonly used in salads, soups, and sushi.

Sissoo Spinach is a leafy green vegetable with small, tender leaves and a mild flavor. It is commonly used in salads, stir-fries, and soups.

Personal Notes and Acknowledgments

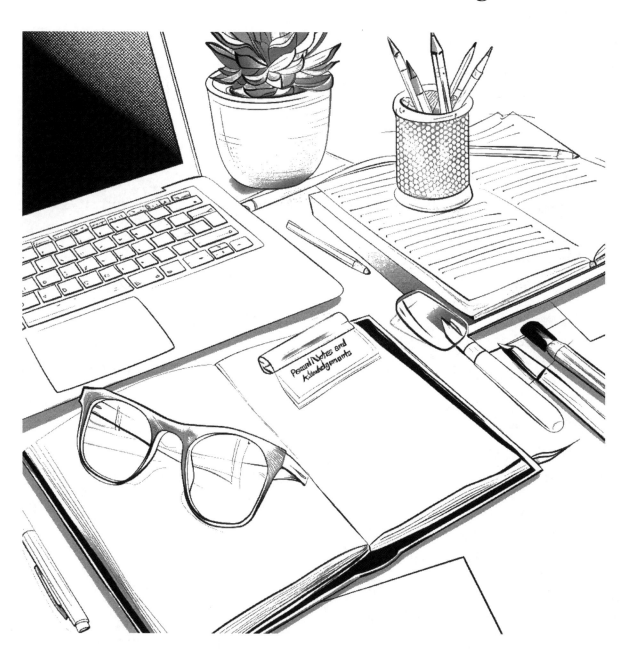

Writing this book has been a labor of love, born out of my journey with diabetes and a desire to share what I've learned along the way. As someone who has lived with the condition for over 15 years, I understand firsthand the challenges and frustrations that come with managing diabetes daily. Through my experiences, I've come to appreciate the importance of making informed dietary choices and finding joy in cooking and eating delicious, nourishing meals.

Acknowledgments:

I want to express my genuine gratitude to everyone who has been by my side throughout the process of writing this book. To my family, friends, and loved ones, thank you for your unwavering encouragement and belief in me. Your support has been invaluable every step of the way.

I am also profoundly grateful to the healthcare professionals who have guided and inspired me on my journey with diabetes. Your expertise and dedication to helping others live healthier lives have been a source of inspiration and motivation for me.

A special thank you to the readers who have embraced this book and found value in its pages. Your feedback and encouragement mean the world to me, and I am humbled by the opportunity to impact your lives positively.

Lastly, I thank the publishing house team for their hard work and dedication in bringing this book to life. Your professionalism and expertise have been instrumental in turning my vision into a reality.

Thank you to everyone who has been a part of this journey. Your support, encouragement, and enthusiasm have made all the difference, and I am grateful beyond words.

Conclusion

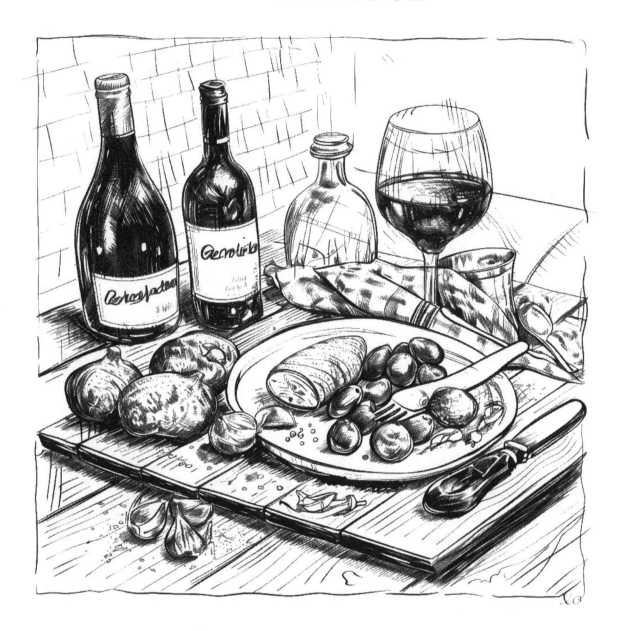

Congratulations on completing this journey through diabetes-friendly recipes and dietary tips! With the knowledge and recipes in this book, you now have the tools to make the right food choices and better manage your diabetes.

Living with diabetes presents unique challenges, but it doesn't have to limit your enjoyment of food or your overall quality of life. As you understand how different foods affect your blood sugar levels, you will begin to make intelligent choices about what you eat; you can take control of your health and well-being.

Throughout this book, we've discussed delicious and nutritious recipes designed to help you maintain stable blood sugar levels while enjoying satisfying meals. From hearty breakfast options to satisfying main dishes and flavorful sauces, there's something for every palate and preference.

One of the fundamental principles we've emphasized is the importance of choosing low-glycemic ingredients. These foods have little effect on blood sugar levels, making them ideal choices for individuals with diabetes. You can maintain more stable blood sugar levels and reduce the risk of complications by incorporating more low-glycemic foods into your diet, such as non-starchy vegetables, whole grains, lean proteins, and healthy fats.

Another critical aspect of managing diabetes is portion control and mindful eating. Pay attention to serving sizes and listen to signs of when your body is hungry and when it is complete. By eating slowly, savoring each bite, and stopping when satisfied, you can avoid overeating and control your blood sugar levels much better.

In addition to focusing on what you eat, paying attention to how you prepare your meals is crucial. Cooking methods that use added fats and sugars, such as grilling, baking, and steaming, are generally healthier for individuals with diabetes. You can prepare delicious and nutritious meals by experimenting with different cooking techniques and flavoring methods.

As you embark on this journey to better health, remember that consistency is critical. Over time, making small and continuous changes to your diet and lifestyle can significantly improve your overall well-being. It's okay to indulge occasionally, but try to balance them with healthier choices most of the time.

Seeking support from healthcare professionals, family, and friends can also be invaluable on your journey to better health. Feel free to reach out for guidance or encouragement whenever you need it. Remember, you're not alone in this journey; resources and support systems are available to help you every step of the way.

I sincerely thank you for choosing this book as a resource for your diabetes-friendly lifestyle. I hope the information and recipes have inspired you to take proactive steps toward better health and wellness. If this book has been helpful to you, please leave a review on Amazon. Your feedback will help people looking for similar resources make informed health decisions.

Thank you once again for your commitment to improving your health and well-being. I wish you all the best on your journey to better health and vitality!

Made in the USA
Columbia, SC
25 August 2024